Approximately 15% of couples experience difficulty in conceiving and a proportion of them may require assisted conception treatment to alleviate continuing infertility. Intrauterine insemination is an effective first line treatment in properly selected cases and is less invasive than in vitro fertilisation and its variants. This multi-author text is a comprehensive account of how to set up and run a successful intrauterine insemination programme. It provides a very practical account and explains clearly the scientific and medical issues. The various chapters deal with design and equipment of the unit, patient selection, counselling, ovarian stimulation strategies, the role of ultrasonography, semen analysis and sperm preparation, intrauterine insemination techniques, semen cryopreservation and banking, and complications. The contributing authors are all experienced practitioners and researchers in reproductive medicine and have created a manual that will be useful to the range of professionals, such as clinicians, andrologists, embryologists, other scientists, nurses, counsellors, psychotherapists and managerial staff, involved in the provision of care for infertile couples. Because of its clear presentation students and patients will also find the volume informative.

# A handbook of intrauterine insemination

# A handbook of intrauterine insemination

Edited by

GODWIN I. MENIRU

*Clinical IVF Consultant, Embryologist and Andrologist,*
*Jerudong Park Medical Centre, Brunei Darussalam*
*Formerly*
*Gynaecologist and Senior Clinical Research Embryologist,*
*London Gynaecology and Fertility Centre*

with the assistance of

PETER R. BRINSDEN

*Medical Director, Bourn Hall Clinic, Cambridgeshire*

IAN L. CRAFT

*Director, London Gynaecology and Fertility Centre*

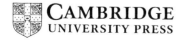

PUBLISHED BY THE PRESS SYNDICATE OF THE UNIVERSITY OF CAMBRIDGE
The Pitt Building, Trumpington Street, Cambridge CB2 1RP, United Kingdom

CAMBRIDGE UNIVERSITY PRESS
The Edinburgh Building, Cambridge CB2 2RU, United Kingdom
40 West 20th Street, New York, NY 10011-4211, USA
10 Stamford Road, Oakleigh, Melbourne 3166, Australia

© Cambridge University Press 1997

This book is in copyright. Subject to statutory exception
and to the provisions of relevant collective licensing agreements,
no reproduction of any part may take place without
the written permission of Cambridge University Press.

First published 1997

Printed in the United Kingdom at the University Press, Cambridge

Typeset in Times New Roman 11/14pt

*A catalogue record for this book is available from the British Library*

*Library of Congress Cataloguing in Publication Data*

A handbook of intrauterine insemination / edited by Godwin I. Meniru,
   Peter R. Brindsen, Ian L. Craft.
     p. cm.
   Includes index.
   ISBN 0 521 58676 3 (pb)
   1. Artificial insemination, Human.   I. Meniru, Godwin I. (Godwin
Ikechukwu), 1960– .   II. Brinsden, Peter R.   III. Craft, Ian L.
(Ian Logan), 1937– .
     [DNLM: 1. Insemination, Artificial.   2. Uterus.   3. Infertility –
therapy.   4. Sperm Banks.   WQ 208 H236 1997]
RG134.H36   1997
618.1′78–dc21
DNLM/DLC   96–39905   CIP
for Library of Congress

ISBN 0 521 58676 3 paperback

Every effort has been made in preparing this book to provide accurate and
up-to-date information which is in accord with accepted standards and practice at
the time of publication. Nevertheless, the authors, editors and publisher can make
no warranties that the information contained herein is totally free from error,
not least because clinincal standards are constantly changing through research and
regulation. The authors, editors and publisher therefore disclaim all liability for
direct or consequential damages resulting from the use of material contained in
this book. The reader is strongly advised to pay careful attention to information
provided by the manufacturer of any drugs or equipment they plan to use.

To all couples who have experienced difficulty in becoming pregnant

# Contents

|  |  |  |
|---|---|---|
| *List of contributors* | | *page* xi |
| *Preface* | | xiii |
| 1 | An overview of intrauterine insemination<br>*Peter R. Brinsden and Samuel F. Marcus* | 1 |
| 2 | Equipment, design and organisation of the unit<br>*Godwin I. Meniru and Susan P. Hutchon* | 9 |
| 3 | Patient selection and management<br>*Godwin I. Meniru and Fidelis T. Akagbosu* | 23 |
| 4 | Fertility counselling<br>*Arlene R. Raeburn and Maryann O. Meniru* | 46 |
| 5 | Ovarian stimulation for the assisted reproduction technologies<br>*Godwin I. Meniru and Ian L. Craft* | 56 |
| 6 | Controlled superovulation for intrauterine insemination<br>*Godwin I. Meniru, Marinos Tsirigotis and Ian L. Craft* | 77 |
| 7 | Ultrasonography in the management of infertility with special reference to intrauterine insemination<br>*Godwin I. Meniru and Ian L. Craft* | 97 |
| 8 | Semen analysis and sperm preparation<br>*Steven D. Fleming, Godwin I. Meniru, Jenny A. Hall and Simon B. Fishel* | 129 |

| | | |
|---|---|---|
| 9 | Intrauterine insemination techniques<br>*Godwin I. Meniru and Peter R. Brinsden* | 146 |
| 10 | The role of the nurse in an insemination programme<br>*Frances E. Bynoe* | 159 |
| 11 | Principles and practice of semen cryopreservation<br>*Steven Green and Steven D. Fleming* | 163 |
| 12 | Donor sperm banking<br>*Joan P. Crich* | 190 |
| 13 | Complications of superovulation and intrauterine insemination<br>*Godwin I. Meniru* | 207 |
| 14 | Concluding remarks: thoughts on the management of infertility<br>*Godwin I. Meniru* | 234 |
| | *Index* | 242 |

# Contributors

**Dr Fidelis T. Akagbosu**, BSc (Hons), MB ChB, MMedSci, FWACS, MFFP, MRCOG
> *Consultant Gynaecologist, Bourn Hall Clinic, Bourn, Cambridge CB3 7TR, UK*

**Mr Peter R. Brinsden**, MB BS, FRCOG
> *Medical Director, Bourn Hall Clinic, Bourn, Cambridge CB3 7TR, UK*

**Mrs Frances E. Bynoe**, SRN, SCM, Certificate in Counselling
> *Infertility Sister, London Gynaecology and Fertility Centre, Cozen's House, 112a Harley Street, London, W1N 1AF, UK*

**Professor Ian L. Craft**, MB BS, FRCS, FRCOG
> *Director, London Gynaecology and Fertility Centre, Cozen's House, 112a Harley Street, London, W1N 1AF, UK*

**Mrs Joan P. Crich**, AIBS
> *Chief MLSO, Department of Histopathology, Nottingham City Hospital Trust, Nottingham NG5 1PB, UK*

**Dr Simon B. Fishel**, BSc, PhD
> *Reader, Department of Obstetrics and Gynaecology; and Scientific Director, Nottingham University Research and Treatment Unit in Reproduction, Queen's Medical Centre, Nottingham NG7 2UH, UK*

**Dr Steven D. Fleming**, BSc, MSc, PhD
> *Lecturer, Department of Obstetrics and Gynaecology, University of Nottingham Queen's Medical Centre, Nottingham NG7 2UH, UK*

**Mr Steven Green**, BSc, MIBiol, CBiol
*Chief Embryologist and PhD Student, Nottingham University Research and Treatment Unit in Reproduction, Department of Obstetrics and Gynaecology, Queen's Medical Centre, Nottingham NG7 2UH, UK*

**Miss Jenny A. Hall**, BSc
*PhD Student, Nottingham University Research and Treatment Unit in Reproduction, Department of Obstetrics and Gynaecology, Queen's Medical Centre, Nottingham NG7 2UH, UK*

**Dr Susan P. Hutchon**, MB ChB, MRCOG
*Clinical Research Fellow, Nottingham University Research and Treatment Unit in Reproduction, Department of Obstetrics and Gynaecology, Queen's Medical Centre, Nottingham NG7 2UH, UK*

**Mr Samuel F. Marcus**, MB BCh, FRCS, MRCOG
*Consultant Gynaecologist, Bourn Hall Clinic, Bourn, Cambridge CB3 7TR, UK*

**Dr Godwin I. Meniru**, MB BS, MMedSci, MFFP, MRCOG
*Clinical IVF Consultant, Embryologist and Andrologist, IVF Unit, Jerudong Park Medical Centre, Jerudong Park 2021, Brunei Darussalam Formerly*
*Gynaecologist and Senior Clinical Research Embryologist, London Gynaecology and Fertility Centre, Cozen's House, 112a Harley Street, London W1N 1AF, UK*

**Mrs Maryann O. Meniru**, BEd, MSc
*Counsellor, Health Psychologist and Lecturer, The Nottingham Trent University, Burton Street, Nottingham NG1 4BU, UK*

**Mrs Arlene R. Raeburn**, BA, Diploma in Counselling
*Infertility Counsellor, Nottingham University Research and Treatment Unit in Reproduction, Department of Obstetrics and Gynaecology, Queen's Medical Centre, Nottingham NG7 2UH, UK*

**Dr Marinos Tsirigotis**, MD, MRCOG
*Gynaecologist, 3 Euripidou Street, Glifada 16674, Athens, Greece*

# Preface

Intrauterine insemination (IUI), with either husband or donor sperm, is now being carried out in an increasing number of units for the management of infertile couples. It is a first line assisted conception treatment method, as well as being one of the least invasive. IUI can therefore be performed outside the confines of sophisticated assisted conception units. Whilst some practitioners will have had the benefit of a formal training programme in this and other aspects of fertility management, many must instead rely on information picked up from diverse sources, which may not necessarily be comprehensive or easy to assimilate and remember. A text such as this is long overdue, as it provides all the basic knowledge required to set up and run an efficient IUI service. Forming a ready source of information that will be useful to beginners and experienced personnel who want to refresh their memory or pick up new ideas and knowledge, this text is presented as a training manual written with the aim of imparting all relevant practical know-how in an easy to read manner. This manual will therefore be valuable to all members of the team, including clinicians, andrologists, embryologists, other scientists, nurses, counsellors and even informed patients.

The handbook begins with a synopsis of IUI and considers its role in the modern management of infertility, followed by a comprehensive account of requirements for establishing a fully functional service. Improper patient selection undermines the efficacy of IUI, thereby obscuring its correct role in infertility management. The criteria for selection as well as contraindications to the treatment are presented together with the actual indications. Counselling has assumed a prominent role in fertility management and general discussion of the current issues in fertility counselling will be followed by the particular requirements of donor insemination. Two chapters deal with the management of the ovarian cycle, which is one of the major determinants of success with assisted conception treatment. The first of these chapters is an historical review of methods of superovulation, while the second deals with drugs and stimulation regimens used specifically for IUI, and the decision process on the timing of insemination. Ultrasound scanning is now used routinely in infertility management and there is a need for a chapter that provides the reader with information on infertility associated pelvic pathologies that are amenable to ultrasound diagnosis. This chapter also deals with ultrasound monitoring of the response to ovarian stimulation, cyclical endometrial activity and the diagnosis of ovulation. Semen analysis is of key importance in patient selection. Following a brief review of sperm preparation methods, two commonly used techniques are presented in an easy to follow manner.

Part of the variability in pregnancy rates following IUI may derive from the multitude of insemination techniques that are currently being used in different centres. Three methods involving different principles will be described as there is presently no agreement on the optimal insemination technique. The nurse is a very important member of the team and her multi-faceted role in the unit is discussed. The advent of effective methods of microassisted fertilisation such as intracytoplasmic sperm injection means that many more infertile men now have a chance of fathering their own child. There is still need for donor insemination and a chapter is devoted to the practical aspects of donor sperm banking. Introduction to cryobiological principles and various methods of semen cryopreservation are presented in an earlier chapter. Although IUI is one of the least invasive of all assisted conception treatments, it still has the potential for complications. The penultimate chapter considers these problems and their management. A personal perspective and proposals for future research in this area make up the last chapter of this manual.

This project has been supported by a panel of experienced workers and well-known authors who are pioneers of various areas in assisted reproduction technology. Every author has been given liberty to adopt an individualised approach to the subject matter but each chapter or section of a chapter, usually starts with a theoretical consideration of the topic followed by a description of the practical aspects. The aim is to provide the readers with a full account of the theoretical basis of the topic and practical issues arising from it. Although controversies abound in this area of assisted conception treatment, we have endeavoured to leave the reader with enough practical information to provide a satisfactory foundation for a successful practice of IUI. At the same time, we have stressed the need for research aimed at gaining more knowledge of prognostic factors. Many thanks to colleagues who have provided perceptive comments and assistance during the preparation of this manual, especially Dr Marinos Tsirigotis. Special thanks go to Dr Simon Fishel, Dr Simon Thornton and Mrs Joan Crich for allowing the use of photographs of equipment in their units and other assistance. Thank you to the team at Cambridge University Press for their foresight and assistance.

GIM
PRB
ILC                                                                                              1997

# 1

# An overview of intrauterine insemination

PETER R. BRINSDEN and SAMUEL F. MARCUS

**Introduction**

The term artificial insemination covers a range of techniques for insemination, which can be performed intravaginally, intracervically, intraperitoneally or intrauterine. Artificial insemination has been used for many years for a number of different indications, and either the husband/partner's or donor sperm may be used. It is almost 200 years since John Hunter advised a man with hypospadias to inject his seminal fluid into his wife's vagina with a syringe, which resulted in a normal pregnancy (Shields 1950). In the nineteenth century, Sims artificially inseminated six women with negative postcoital tests. He used their husbands' semen obtained from the vagina after intercourse; one pregnancy was achieved (Sims 1886). The first reported case of human donor insemination was by William Pankhurst in 1884 in Philadelphia, USA (Hard 1909).

The rationale for the use of intrauterine insemination (IUI) is to reduce the effect of factors such as vaginal acidity and cervical mucus hostility and to benefit from the deposition a bolus of concentrated motile morphologically normal sperm as close as possible to the oocytes. Sperm preparation methods developed for in vitro fertilisation (IVF) and embryo transfer (ET), such as the wash and swim-up technique and the use of Percoll gradients (Percoll; Pharmacia LKB Biotechnology, Uppsala, Sweden), have led to a resurgence of interest in IUI. Consequently many workers in the field of infertility are now using this experience to perform IUI with washed motile capacitated sperm (Sher *et al.* 1984; Sun *et al.* 1987; Yovich & Matson 1988), making this a frequently used first choice of the assisted conception techniques that may be used for the treatment of infertile women with patent fallopian tubes. The use of washed prepared sperm for IUI has resulted in a significant reduction in the side-effects associated with the use of neat semen for IUI, such as painful uterine cramps, collapse and infection (Allen *et al.* 1985; Yovich & Matson 1988; Golan *et al.* 1989).

**Methods of insemination**

Intrauterine insemination may be carried out in either a natural or stimulated cycle. Many ovarian stimulation protocols have been devised for use with IUI, including clomiphene citrate alone or in combination with gonadotrophins and human chorionic gonadotrophin (hCG), gonadotrophins alone or combined with the use of a gonadotrophin releasing hormone agonist and hCG. The rationale for the use of superovulation with IUI is to increase the number of oocytes available for insemination and thus the chance of implantation occurring. Stimulation also increases steroid production, which may in turn improve the chance of fertilisation and embryo implantation (Wallach 1991). When considering whether to use ovarian stimulation for IUI, the benefit of increased success rates achieved compared with natural cycles must be balanced against the increased cost of medication and monitoring as well as the potential side-effects of these medications, including ovarian hyperstimulation syndrome, and the increased incidence of maternal and neonatal complications associated with multiple pregnancies (Sheldon *et al.* 1988; Levene *et al.* 1989; Lipitz *et al.* 1990).

There are several methods for timing ovulation in natural or stimulated cycles, including simple methods such as the measurement of basal body temperature, found to be the least accurate, and assessment of cyclical changes to the cervical mucus. Templeton *et al.* (1982) showed that in 35% of cycles the optimum mucus score was observed the day before the luteinizing hormone (LH) surge, in 44% of cycles it was optimum on the day of the LH surge and in 18% of cycles on the day after the LH surge, while in 3% it occurred 2 days after the LH surge. More recently, the detection of the serum or urinary LH surge and ultrasound assessment of follicular growth and rupture have proved to be the most accurate methods of monitoring cycles. Vermesh *et al.* (1987) showed that using a dipstick LH test kit predicted ovulation in 84% of cycles in his series. In a stimulated cycle, if hCG is administered when the average diameter of the leading follicle is 20 mm, rupture of the follicle may be expected 34–40 hours later (O'Herlihy *et al.* 1982).

The ideal sperm preparation technique is the one which will achieve the largest number of morphologically normal motile spermatozoa in a small volume of physiological culture medium free from seminal plasma, leucocytes and bacteria (Pardo & Bancells 1989). Although there is no threshold of sperm concentration below which pregnancy is impossible, most conceptions occur when the concentration of inseminated motile sperm is more than one million per millilitre. The degree of motility and percentage of morphologically normal spermatozoa are the most important variables in fertility prognosis. There are several different sperm preparation techniques for IUI; each has its own advantages and disadvantages (Berger *et al.* 1985). Sperm preparation using the Percoll gradient technique yields the highest number of motile spermatozoa when compared with simple washing or swim-up methods, and the Percoll technique significantly reduces bacterial contamination (Punjabi *et al.* 1990). The manufacturer of Percoll has recently stated that Percoll should not be used for sperm preparation in human assisted conception treatment. Alternative density gradient centrifugation media will be discussed in a later chapter.

**Indications**

Couples seeking artificial insemination should be fully evaluated, including a complete medical history, a clinical examination and investigation for the presence of any abnormality such as tubal damage or ovulatory disorder. It is also essential that couples receive adequate counselling prior to starting treatment, especially when donor sperm is to be used. Couples should also be assured of complete confidentiality, and informed of the means by which donors are selected and matched, the cost of treatment, the probability of success, complications and, in the UK when using donor sperm, the regulations imposed by the Human Fertilisation and Embryology Authority (HFEA).

The main indications for donor insemination are gross male subfertility (azoospermia or severe oligoasthenoteratozoospermia), familial or genetic disease such as Huntington's disease, haemophilia and also severe Rhesus isoimmunisation. The use of cryopreserved semen in donor insemination programmes is now mandatory in most countries to minimise the possibility of transmission of the human immunodeficiency virus to the recipients.

The introduction of oocyte–sperm micromanipulation procedures such as intracytoplasmic sperm injection (ICSI) into IVF-ET programmes (Palermo *et al.* 1992), has made it possible to achieve fertilisation and pregnancies when only very few spermatozoa are available. Prior to the development of techniques such as microepididymal sperm aspiration (Tournaye *et al.* 1994), percutaneous epididymal sperm aspiration (Craft *et al.* 1995) and more recently testicular sperm extraction (Silber *et al.* 1995), men with bilateral congenital absence of the vas deferens, surgically unreconstructable vasa or other causes of vasal obstruction had very little chance of fathering their own children. Now, however, if these techniques are combined with ICSI, they can be offered a real chance of achiev-

Table 1.1. *Indications for insemination with husband's/partner's semen*

| 1. | Ejaculatory failure | – anatomical (e.g. hypospadias)<br>– neurological (e.g. spinal cord injury)<br>– retrograde ejaculation<br>– psychological (e.g. impotence) |
|---|---|---|
| 2. | Cervical factor | – cervical mucus hostility<br>– poor cervical mucus |
| 3. | Male subfertility | – oligozoospermia<br>– asthenozoospermia<br>– teratozoospermia<br>– oligoasthenoteratozoospermia |
| 4. | Immunological | – male antisperm antibodies<br>– female antisperm antibodies (cervical, serum) |
| 5. | Idiopathic infertility | |
| 6. | Endometriosis | – mild, moderate |
| 7. | Some cases with combined infertility factors | |

ing paternity with their own sperm (Devroey *et al.* 1995; Sherman *et al.* 1995). These methods have reduced the demand for donor insemination, but the cost of these procedures puts them beyond the means of many couples.

Ejaculatory failure is the classical indication for IUI using husband's semen (Table 1.1), because of the inability of the partner to ejaculate into the vagina, while cervical mucus hostility is a logical indication as the insemination method bypasses the cervical canal. The most common indications for IUI are for some of the less severe forms of male factor infertility and for unexplained infertility, and yet these are the most controversial. Other indications for IUI are some immunological causes of infertility and mild to moderate endometriosis.

## Results and factors affecting success rates

The results of IUI in terms of pregnancy rates per treatment cycle vary considerably between clinics and evaluation of the results is difficult because of the heterogeneity of the patient population and the different ovarian stimulation protocols used in the studies. Although there are a large number of published studies on IUI, most of these are retrospective and/or on small numbers; only a few are prospective and randomised trials. There is an undoubted need for a large prospective randomised study to evaluate the real effectiveness of IUI and to elicit which group of patients will benefit most from this treatment.

Table 1.2. *Pregnancy success rates for intrauterine insemination related to the cause of infertility*

| Indication | Martinez et al. (1993) | Crosignani et al. (1991); Crosignani & Walters (1994) | Bourn Hall Clinic (1989–93) |
|---|---|---|---|
| Idiopathic infertility | 18 (0–40) | 27 (0–67) | 12.3 |
| Cervical mucus hostility | 14 (5–29) | | 16.4 |
| Immunological infertility | 10 (3–18) | | 10.0 |
| Endometriosis | 11 (0–18) | | 0 |
| Male subfertility | 10 (0–20) | 12.8 (0–40) | 21.0 |
| Ejaculatory failure | 11 (0–18) | | 13.3 |
| Combined factors | | | 15.8 |

*Notes:*
Values are % (range)

Table 1.2 summarises the results of some published series on IUI treatment and our own unpublished retrospective data from 237 patients having 452 treatment cycles. The European Society of Human Reproduction and Embryology (ESHRE) Multi-Centre Prospective Study (Crosignani et al. 1991), compared ovulation induction alone with ovulation induction in conjunction with IUI, intraperitoneal insemination (IPI), gamete intra-fallopian transfer (GIFT) and IVF in the treatment of unexplained infertility. The pregnancy rate achieved from superovulation alone was less than when combined with IUI, IPI, GIFT or IVF. The ESHRE Multi-Centre Trial (Crosignani & Walters 1994), which compared ovulation induction alone and ovulation induction combined with IUI, IPI, GIFT and IVF in the treatment of male subfertility, showed that ovulation induction with IUI, GIFT and IVF gave better results than IPI and ovulation induction alone.

Martinez et al. (1993), in an extensive review of the literature from 1980 to 1991, showed that there was marked variation in the results of IUI between different clinics. Remohi et al. (1989) reported a series of 489 cycles of controlled ovarian stimulation and IUI. The cycle fecundity rate was 0.07 for the first four cycles and 0.03 for the fifth through tenth cycle. In this series 94% of the pregnancies occurred in the first four attempts. Other retrospective analyses of IUI data (Martinez et al. 1988; Roger et al. 1988; Wallach 1991), using life-table analysis showed a relatively constant probability of becoming pregnant after each IUI treatment through six cycles, and thereafter is hardly increased by continuing for longer. Most clinicians are agreed that further evaluation and discussion of the other treatment options available to couples should be carried out with them after four to six cycles of IUI.

A live birth rate of 6.5% per donor insemination treatment cycle for the UK is reported in the Annual Report of the HFEA (1995). This report was based on data from licenced donor insemination clinics in 1993. There is a wide variation of results between clinics, ranging from 0 to 42.6%. The multiple pregnancy rate also varied from 0 to 50%, with a triplet pregnancy rate of between 0 and 25%. Our own results during the same time period gave a live birth rate of 17.4%, with a 10% twin rate and no triplets.

### Complications of treatment

There are few complications to treatment by IUI; failure of the treatment could be said to be the most frequent. The complication which causes couples the most concern is the possibility of using the wrong semen sample. Other complications include the possibility of transmission of venereal disease and the remote possibility of consanguineous insemination when using donor sperm. Uterine contractions, intrauterine infection and anaphylaxis may also occur, especially if neat semen is used, which it should never be. Finally, the chances of ovarian hyperstimulation from the drugs used for ovulation induction, and multiple pregnancy should also be considered as possible complications of treatment; these can be minimised by careful monitoring of treatment cycles.

### Conclusion

Intrauterine insemination is an effective, non-invasive, relatively simple and cheap method of treatment. It can be provided more easily to more infertile couples in district general hospitals than can the more specialised techniques such as IVF provided there are adequate facilities for semen preparation and cycle monitoring. Careful selection of patients is important. Those who will benefit most are young women with patent fallopian tubes, with no ovulatory disorder, no endometriosis of moderate or severe degree and no severe degree of male factor infertility in their partner. All couples require in-depth advice and counselling about the method, the effectiveness and the complications of treatment.

Although the main advantage of IUI over IVF is its simplicity, there are many advantages of IVF over IUI, principally a higher pregnancy rate, the knowledge obtained about fertilisation of oocytes and the ability to cryopreserve any spare embryos that may result from a treatment cycle. IVF or ICSI are the only realistic treatments for couples with severe male factor infertility, and IVF for severe endometriosis and infertility due to severe tubal damage. Although IUI can be performed outside of specialist units, a clinic with IVF facilities offers the best setting in case complications such as ovarian hyperstimulation syndrome occur, as patients can be offered the chance to convert to IVF and the possibility of freezing any surplus embryos.

## References

Allen M. C., Herbert I., Maxson W. S., Rogers B. J., Diamond M. A. & Wentz A.C. (1985) Intrauterine insemination: a critical review. *Fertility and Sterility* **44**, 569–580.

Berger T., Marrs R. P. & Moyer D. L. (1985) Comparison of techniques for selection of motile spermatozoa. *Fertility and Sterility* **43**, 268–273.

Craft I. L., Khalifa Y., Boulos A., Pelekanos M., Foster C. & Tsirigotis M. (1995) Factors influencing the outcome of in-vitro fertilization with percutaneous aspirated epididymal spermatozoa and intracytoplasmic sperm injection in azoospermic men. *Human Reproduction* **10**, 1791–1794.

Crosignani P. G. & Walters D. E. (1994) Clinical pregnancy and male subfertility, the ESHRE multicentre trial on the treatment of male subfertility. *Human Reproduction* **9**, 1112–1118.

Crosignani P. G., Walters D. E. & Soliani A. (1991) The ESHRE multicentre trial on the treatment of unexplained infertility: a preliminary report. *Human Reproduction* **6**, 953–958.

Devroey P., Nagy Z., Goossens A., Tournaye H., Camus M., Van Steirteghem A. C. & Silber S. J. (1995) Pregnancies after testicular sperm extraction and intracytoplasmic sperm injection in non-obstructive azoospermia. *Human Reproduction* **6**, 1457–1460.

Golan A., Ron-El R. & Herman A. (1989) Ovarian hyperstimulation syndrome. An update review. *Obstetrical and Gynecological Survey* **44**, 430–440.

Hard A. D. (1909) Artificial impregnation. *Medical World* **27**, 253.

Human Fertilisation and Embryology Authority. (1995) *Human Fertilisation and Embryology Authority: 4th Annual Report*, 4th edition, London.

Levene M. I., Wild J. & Steer P. (1989) Higher multiple births and the modern management of infertility in Britain. *British Journal of Obstetrics and Gynaecology* **99**, 607–613.

Lipitz S., Fishel S., Watts C., Ben-Rafael Z., Barkai G. & Reichman B. (1990) High order multifetal gestation – management and outcome. *Obstetrics and Gynecology* **76**, 215–218.

Martinez A. R., Bernardus R. E. & Vermeiden J. P. W. (1988) Factors affecting pregnancy results after intrauterine insemination (Abstr.). Presented at the 4th Meeting of the European Society of Human Reproduction and Embryology Barcelona, Spain July 3–6 1988. *Human Reproduction* Abstract 35.

Martinez A. R., Bernardus R. E., Vermeiden J. P. W. & Schoemaker J. (1993) Basic questions on intrauterine insemination: an update. *Obstetrical and Gynecological Survey* **48**, 811–828.

O'Herlihy C., Pepperell R. J. & Robinson H. P. (1982) Ultrasound timing of human chorionic gonadotrophin administration in clomiphene stimulated cycles. *Obstetrics and Gynecology* **59**, 40–45.

Palermo G., Joris H., Devroey P. & Van Steirtegheim A. C. (1992) Pregnancies after intracytoplasmic injection of single spermatozoa into an oocyte. *Lancet* **340**, 17–18.

Pardo M. & Bancells N. (1989) Artificial insemination with husband's sperm (AIH). Techniques for sperm selection. *Archives of Andrology* **22**, 15–27.

Punjabi V., Gerris J., Van Bijilen J., Delbeke L., Giles M. & Buytaert P. (1990) Comparison between different pre-treatment techniques for sperm recovery prior to intrauterine insemination, GIFT or IVF. *Human Reproduction* **5**, 75–78.

Remohi J., Gastaldi C., Patrizio P., Gerli S., Ord T., Asch R. H. & Balmaceda J. (1989) Intrauterine insemination and controlled ovarian hyperstimulation in cycles before GIFT. *Human Reproduction* **4**, 918–920.

Roger A., Lalich D. O., Edward L., Marut M. D., Gail S., Prins P. & Scommergna A. (1988) Life table analyses of intrauterine insemination pregnancy rates. *American Journal of Obstetrics and Gynecology* **158**, 980–984.

Sheldon R., Kemmann E., Bohrer M. & Pasquale S. (1988) Multiple gestation is associated with the use of high sperm numbers in the intrauterine insemination specimen in women undergoing gonadotrophin stimulation. *Fertility and Sterility* **49**, 607–610.

Sher G., Knutzen V. K., Stratton C. J., Montakhab M. & Allenson S. (1984) *In vitro* sperm capacitation and transcervical intrauterine insemination for the treatment of refractory infertility. *Fertility and Sterility* **41**, 260–264.

Sherman J., Silber S. J., Nagy Z., Liu J., Tournaye H., Lissens W., Ferec C., Liebaers I., Devroey P. & Van Steirtegheim A. C. (1995) The use of epididymal and testicular spermatozoa for intracytoplasmic sperm injection: the genetic implication for male infertility. *Human Reproduction* **10**, 2031–2043.

Shields F.E. (1950) Artificial insemination as related to females. *Fertility and Sterility* **1**, 271–280.

Silber S. J., Van Steirtegheim A. C., Liu J., Nagy Z., Tournaye H. & Devroey P. (1995) High fertilization and pregnancy rates after intracytoplasmic sperm injection with spermatozoa obtained from testicle biopsy. *Human Reproduction* **10**, 148–152.

Sims J. M. (1886) *Clinical notes on uterine surgery with special reference to the management of the sterile condition.* London: Harolwiche.

Sun S. L., Gastaldi C., Paterson E., Maza L. M. & Stone S. C. (1987) Comparison of techniques for selection of bacteria-free sperm preparations. *Fertility and Sterility* **48**, 659–663.

Templeton A. A., Penney G. C. & Lees M. M. (1982) Relation between the luteinizing hormone peak, the nadir of basal body temperature and the cervical mucus score. *British Journal of Obstetrics and Gynaecology* **89**, 985–988.

Tournaye H., Devroey P., Liu P., Nagy Z., Lissens W. & Van Steirtegheim A. C. (1994) Microsurgical epididymal sperm aspiration and intraycytoplasmic sperm injection: a new effective approach to infertility as a result of congenital bilateral absence of the vas deferens. *Fertility and Sterility* **62**, 644–647.

Vermesh M., Kletzky O. A., Davajam V. & Israel, R. (1987) Monitoring techniques to predict and detect ovulation. *Fertility and Sterility* **47**, 259–264.

Wallach E. E. (1991) Gonadotrophin treatment of the ovulatory patient: the pros and cons of empiric therapy for infertility. *Fertility and Sterility* **55**, 478–480.

Yovich J. L. & Matson P. L. (1988) The treatment of infertility by the high intrauterine insemination of the husband's washed spermatozoa. *Human Reproduction* **3**, 939–943.

# 2

# Equipment, design and organisation of the unit

GODWIN I. MENIRU and SUSAN P. HUTCHON

**Introduction**

What the unit layout, type and location of equipment as well as management issues should be are very important considerations which have to be addressed at the planning stages of an intrauterine insemination (IUI) service and they depend on local circumstances. IUI could be one of a range of treatments being offered in an assisted conception unit. No separate requirements are needed in such a centre as appropriate equipment, manpower and drugs are already in place and being used for other assisted conception treatments. A unit may start off initially with IUI as the only procedure being offered and later on commence other treatments. In this case, initial planning and equipment of the unit should take long-term goals into consideration. IUI can also be performed as an office procedure by the gynaecologist in private practice who may use facilities in nearby hospitals for follicular tracking, sperm preparation and management of complications in patients.

There is an increasing trend in general or teaching hospital gynaecological units for consultants with special interests in fertility management to introduce an IUI service into the department. Laboratory and ultrasound scanning facilities are often shared with the rest of the Gynaecology Department and indeed the whole hospital. Scheduling problems may be encountered as no priority will be given for access of infertility patients to facilities such as ultrasound scanning especially at short notice. The ultrasonographer may not have experience in follicular tracking which may influence the standard of care. Semen preparation in a general laboratory is not ideal because of the real risk of contamination from the myriad biological specimens and toxic chemicals that are present there. These drawbacks are being highlighted not to condemn IUI in such hospitals but to indicate the need for dedicated facilities which should be the aim in any serious unit as soon as the patient throughput increases to the point where it justifies the capital expenditure involved.

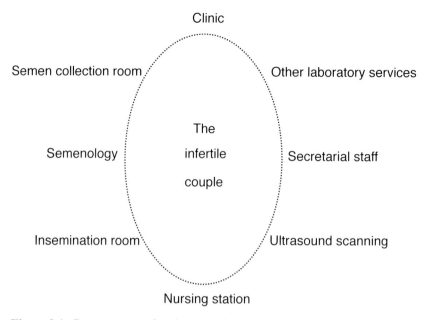

Figure 2.1. Components of an intrauterine insemination service.

The following section will consider specific requirements for an IUI service (Figure 2.1) which may have to be tailored to fit peculiar circumstances obtaining in any particular location. Most instruments and supplies have more than one manufacturer and model. The specific brand to be used depends on cost considerations, preference of scientific and medical personnel, nearness to manufacturers and availability of after-sales training and maintenance services. For this reason, generic, not brand names, will be used as much as possible in the following account.

### Semen collection room

A room should be provided for the production and collection of semen. This room is ideally located in a quiet part of the unit. Privacy is reinforced by hanging a 'DO NOT DISTURB' sign on the door when the room is in use. Alternatively, it could be left unmarked so as to avoid drawing unnecessary attention to it as this may precipitate what it was meant to prevent. The room should be comfortable, large enough to accommodate two people, usually the man's partner, and furnished with any materials thought necessary to aid production of semen such as magazines and video films.

Table 2.1. *Instrumentation for the semenology laboratory*

| | |
|---|---|
| Pipette controller | Liquid nitrogen cylinder |
| Carbon dioxide cylinders | Micropipettor |
| Centrifuge | Multiple bank totalising counters |
| Computer (networked preferably) | Refrigerator |
| Fyrite or Draeger tube | Single tally counter |
| Incubator | Slide warmer |
| Phase contrast light microscope | Sperm counting chamber |
| Class 2 cabinet | Spirit burners |
| Liquid nitrogen dewars | Test tube rack |

## Semenology facilities

### *Personnel*

If patient numbers in a General or Teaching Hospital justify employing a semenologist this will be the best option but it is more likely that the hospital laboratory scientist who carries out the routine semen analyses will have to perform this duty. Competence in semen preparation should not be assumed. In addition to studying the relevant texts a short period of intensive training should be arranged at the nearby assisted conception unit. The semenologist can then continue to improve his or her skills with semen samples sent in for routine analysis till he/she becomes competent to prepare samples for clinical use. The need for accurate and reproducible techniques should be stressed as data emanating from here forms the basis for most audit and research in the unit.

### *Hardware*

Basic equipment requirements are shown in Table 2.1 and Figures 2.2–2.8. Detailed directions for their use can be found in accompanying product manuals and technical support should be available from these manufacturers who usually arrange for demonstration and on-site training following their installation. Extended warranty and maintenance contracts should be arranged at the outset as many of these instruments will require regular servicing and repair. On arrival at the laboratory the semen sample is left on the bench if semen analysis is the only procedure to be carried out. If however sperm preparation is also to be carried out, the container is placed in the laminar flow hood where all the relevant work except centrifugation and microscopy, is subsequently carried out. The Class II type cabinet is now

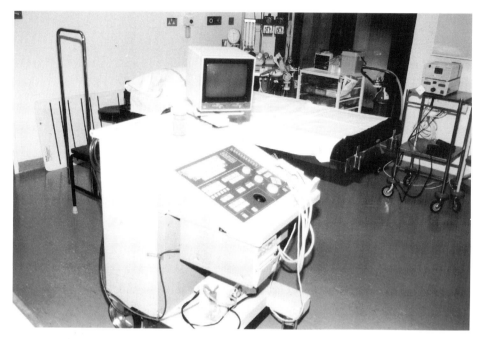

Figure 2.2. Ultrasound scanning equipment and examination couch with adjustable sections. Both vaginal and abdominal transducers must be available.

recommended in order to reduce the chances of infection to staff from specimens that are being handled. Previously, the filtered air from the laminar flow hood cabinets blew directly towards the user of the cabinet. The Class II type cabinet however directs the stream of filtered air downwards. The working surface of the laminar flow hood is wiped down with 70% ethanol at the beginning of each working day. Special plastic bags and 'sharps-safe' bins are provided for laboratory and clinical wastes and these are sealed and removed when full or at the end of each working day.

Spillage is wiped off with dry paper towels. Should it become necessary to use detergents or alcohol it is best to wait till work on the current sample has been completed before doing so. At the end of each day, the room is cleaned together with the work surfaces and instruments. Unused supplies are put away while partially used ones are either disposed of or re-sterilised, depending on their nature and manufacturers' instructions. Regular microbiological screening of the work environment is required to ensure continued absence of pathogenic micro-organisms. Swabs are taken from all areas of the laboratory including air vents.

A bench centrifuge with swing-out rotor is a necessity and should be calibrated in $\times g$ rather than revolutions per minute. An incubator is also impor-

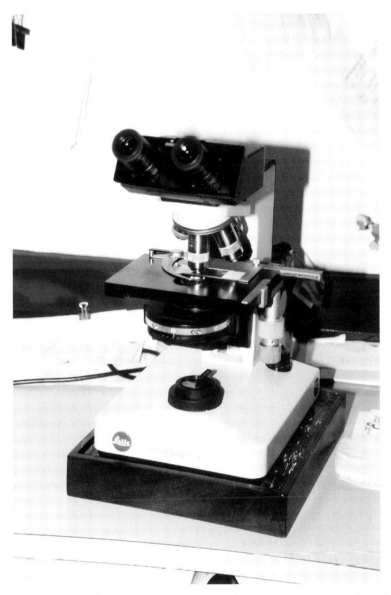

Figure 2.3. A phase contrast microscope is an important piece of equipment in a semenology laboratory.

tant and attempts have to be made to acquire one for sole use by the semenologist. Sperm preparations and equilibrating culture media are maintained at 37 °C and locks should be fitted on the incubator for security purposes. Sophisticated models incorporating a self-adjusting flow of carbon dioxide ($CO_2$) and humidification chambers cost more but they are also more convenient to use. A 100% $CO_2$ gas cylinder is connected to the incubator with a

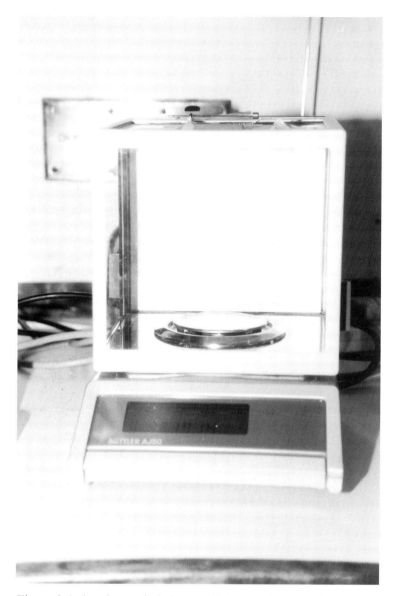

Figure 2.4. An electronic balance will be required if culture medium or cryoprotectants are made in the laboratory.

millipore filter being placed along the pipe that leads to the incubator in order to remove any particulate material including bacteria. Units on a tight budget can still achieve excellent results using ordinary incubators; however, containers of culture media need to be gassed directly from 5% $CO_2$-in-air cylinders and closed tightly before being placed in the incubator. The same applies to sperm preparations. It is prudent for manufacturer's certificates confirming the

*Equipment, design and unit organisation*

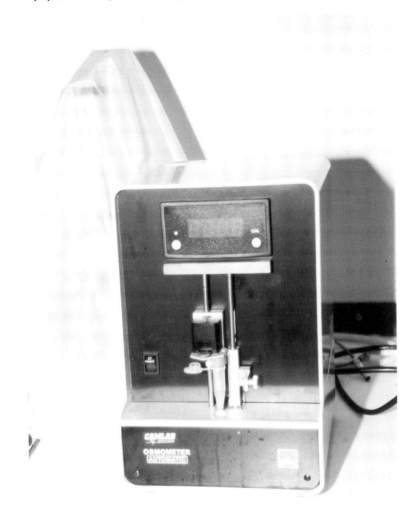

Figure 2.5. There should be access to an osmometer if culture medium or cryoprotectants are made or modified in the laboratory. The greater the throughput of treatment cycles in the unit, the greater the need for an in-house osmometer.

composition of the gas mixture to be insisted upon for every cylinder supplied (S. Fishel; personal communication).

Dewars and liquid nitrogen cylinders will only be required if frozen semen is kept in the laboratory. Some patients may require donor semen, so a dewar

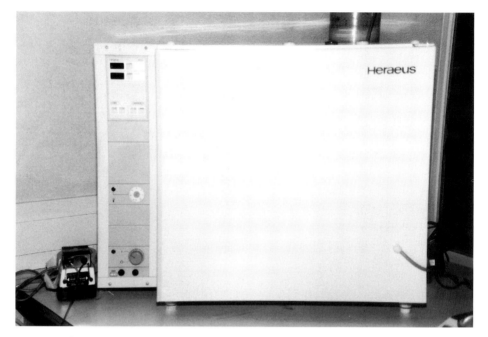

Figure 2.6. It is convenient to use a humidifying incubator capable of maintaining a 5% carbon dioxide-in-air mixture. Regular cleaning and disinfection should however be carried out to prevent overgrowth by bacteria and fungi.

specifically made for transporting frozen specimens should be available in the unit although a nearby sperm bank can use their own in supplying required samples to the unit. Donor sperm banking and insemination will be discussed in a later chapter. Use of the Makler sperm counting chamber (Sefi-Medical Instruments Ltd, Haifa, Israel) is highly recommended because of its accuracy. The binocular phase contrast microscope should have ×10, ×20, ×40 and ×100 objectives and ×10 eyepiece. It is preferable to have a microscope with a integral or fitted heated stage which is kept at 37 °C. The semenologist should have access to a fume cupboard for handling chemicals such as the xylene-based Xam neutral medium (BDH Laboratory Supplies, Poole, UK) which is used in gluing coverslips onto slides.

*Consumables*

Consumables used in the laboratory include those listed in Table 2.2. It is more convenient and safer to use disposable items, which are bought already sterilised and tested for toxicity to sperms. Several culture media have been used by different workers and none of them seem to have any advantage over the other in so far as sperm preparation and culture are concerned. A simple medium

*Equipment, design and unit organisation*

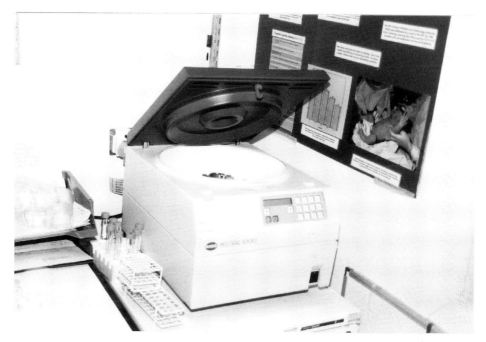

Figure 2.7. A centrifuge with swing-out rotor and calibrated in x *g* is preferred to one with a fixed rotor calibrated only in revolutions per minute.

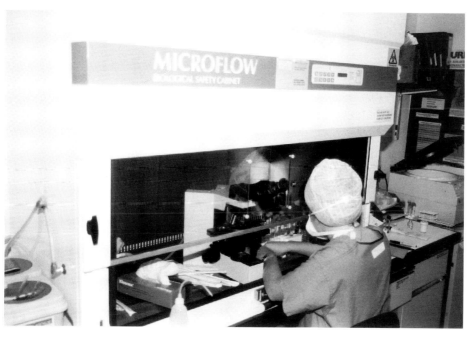

Figure 2.8. A Class 2 safety cabinet reduces contamination of semen samples as well as affording some protection to staff.

Table 2.2. *'Consumables' required in the laboratory*

---

100% PureSperm (Scandinavian IVF Science AB, Gothenburg, Sweden)
19G hypodermic needle
50 ml polystyrene tissue culture flasks for equilibrating culture medium
70% ethanol and water washbottles
70% ethanol impregnated tissue wipes
Albumin Human Immuno 200mg/ml (Medi-Cult, Denmark)
Centrifuge tubes with conical base (5 and 13ml)
Crystapen 600mg (Britannia Pharmaceuticals, Surrey, UK)
Earle's balanced salt solution (Sigma Chemical Co., St. Louis, USA)
Coloured adhesive tape with dispenser for labelling centrifuge tubes
Microscope coverslips
Microscope slides
Pasteur pipettes (pre-plugged and pre-sterilised)
Permanent marker pen
Pippette tips
Plastic syringes (1, 5, 10 and 20ml) without rubber components
Polystyrene pipettes (1, 5 and 10ml)
Powder-free latex rubber gloves
Pyruvic acid (Sigma Chemical Co., St. Louis, USA)
Rubber droppers for Pasteur pipettes
'Sharps-safe' bin
Stationary (including record forms)
Tissue paper
Water (Analar, BDH Laboratory Supplies, Poole, England)

---

such as Earle's balanced salt solution supplemented with protein, pyruvate and antibiotic is quite satisfactory and relatively inexpensive.

### Health And Safety

Health and safety rules must be observed and protective attire (Table 2.3) worn as every semen sample is a potential source of infection to staff and other patients. Care should be exercised when handling thawing glass ampoules of cryopreserved semen as they may explode. Do not leave equipment lying carelessly around because they may become damaged, contaminated or cause injury to staff. Appropriate texts should be consulted for more details (WHO 1992; Mortimer 1994). The responsibility for safeguarding the health of all those who have access to the unit rests on everyone. Safety handbooks should be issued to every new member of staff and appropriate warning signs are dis-

Table 2.3. *Safe practice in the laboratory*

Face masks
Gloves
Caps
Spectacles/goggles
Laboratory coats
First aid equipment
Irrigation fluid for the eye
Regular handwashing
Disposable laboratory supplies

Table 2.4. *Requirements for insemination*

| | |
|---|---|
| Cotton wool swabs | Paper hand towel |
| Cusco's speculum | Patient drape |
| Gallipot | Normal saline |
| Gauze swabs | Sanitary towel (Not tampon) |
| Syringes (1, 5, 20ml) | Drapes |
| Insemination devices | Powder-free gloves |
| Kidney dish | Tenaculum |
| Non-toothed dissecting forceps | |

played in prominent areas of the unit. Safe working practices should be stressed and those who do not keep to the rules should be corrected. All accidents should be reported immediately.

Prohibited activities in the laboratory include smoking, eating, drinking, and applying cosmetics. In other words, nothing should be put into the mouth while in the laboratory. Gloves should be worn while handling biological specimens, and safety glasses too. Materials should be disposed of correctly and any spillage wiped off immediately. It is advisable to centrifuge in sealed containers. All tenets of COSHH (Control of Substances Hazardous to Health) and GLP (Good Laboratory Practice) must be adhered to.

### Ultrasound scanning

Follicular development is monitored with serial ultrasound scans performed usually with a transvaginal probe at a frequency of 5–7.5 MHz. A thermal printer provides a hard copy of ultrasound scan findings but this is not usually required in routine follicular scanning. The timing and intervals between scans depend on the protocol of ovarian stimulation being used and other factors such as patient response patterns and the appearance of complications. Serial hormone assay is not necessary for monitoring ovarian stimulation for assisted conception treatment (Golan *et al.* 1994) and has not been used in our programme since it started in 1976 (Tsirigotis *et al.* 1995). This policy is compatible with normal pregnancy rates and a low incidence of ovarian hyperstimulation syndrome.

### Nursing station

Staffing requirements depend on the scope and volume of the clinical workload. At least one full-time nurse should be employed and designated Infertility Sister. Apart from specific clinical duties she acts as a liaison between the patient and other personnel of the service. Patients also contact her at different stages during evaluation and treatment to arrange hospital appointments. She needs to be knowledgeable about gynaecological and especially fertility disorders because it is likely that patients would discuss some aspects of their management with her. The nursing station may be set up for counselling, injecting, teaching patients self-injecting and administrative work. The role of nurses in an intrauterine insemination programme will be discussed in a later chapter.

### Outpatient clinic facilities and insemination room

A room is made available within the complex for consultations between medical staff and patients. Insemination of patients may take place here but as current techniques require that the patient lies on the couch for sometime afterwards, it may be more appropriate to have another room for insemination. Normal clinic furnishings and equipment are suitable but the couch must be adjustable so as to allow placement of the patient in a slight head down tilt after insemination. Instruments required for insemination are listed in Table 2.4. The Wallace insemination catheter (H. G. Wallace Ltd, Colchester, UK) is usually adequate but some Frydman's catheters (Laboratoire CCD, Paris, France) should be made available for use in cases where difficulty is experienced with passing the catheter through the cervical os. Other insemination devices and techniques will be described in Chapter 9.

## Other staff and requirements

An assisted conception unit will normally have Medical and Scientific Directors while a Consultant Gynaecologist heads the General/Teaching Hospital IUI service. Supporting medical staff include junior colleagues and research fellows who most probably have additional duties in other sections of the Gynaecology Department. The extent of involvement of these staff in various aspects of the work in the unit will vary according to their interests and specific characteristics of the unit. There is no reason why serial ultrasound monitoring of ovarian response to superovulation, semen analysis and sperm preparation cannot be performed by medical staff within the Gynaecology Department as these skills can be acquired easily. The tendency to leave inexperienced and junior staff to work unsupervised in the IUI service, however, should be avoided because this may compromise the efficacy of the treatment being offered. IUI is equally as important as in vitro fertilisation (IVF) and related techniques. Furthermore, IUI has many attributes that make it a desirable alternative to IVF.

Secretarial staff may be shared with the rest of the unit or department. Networked computer terminals are normal features of certain units and absent in others. Current trends involve the use of a customised database software package with data being entered prospectively from various terminals in the unit. In so doing repetition of tasks is avoided and patient information is available to unit personnel who directly access the database after logging in with their assigned password. Further benefits of such a setup will be realised during research and audit activities.

## Conclusion

A universal blueprint for an IUI service is neither possible nor necessary due to the great variability that will, as a consequence of human nature, exist in most units. An attempt has however been made to describe the basic conditions that have to be fulfilled for the establishment of an efficient outfit. Other issues such as hours of duty, unit rota and weekend work depend on local conditions and the availability of staff. It must be stressed however that there is need for continuous cover for patient management even outside normal working hours. Thus key members of staff have to be present for a few hours during the weekend in order to carry out ultrasound scans, administer gonadotrophin injections, carry out sperm preparation and insemination because it is only through this that the best chance of success is given to each treatment cycle. The addition of gonadotrophin releasing hormone agonists to superovulation regimens, however, may lighten the weekend workload because ovulation can be programmed to occur during weekdays.

### Acknowledgement

We thank Drs Simon Fishel and Simon Thornton for the photographs used in this chapter.

### References

Golan A., Herman A., Soffer Y., Bukovsky I. & Ron-El R. (1994) Ultrasonic control without hormone determination for ovulation induction in in-vitro fertilization/embryo transfer with gonadotrophin-releasing hormone analogue and human menopausal gonadotrophin. *Human Reproduction* **9**, 1631–1633.

Mortimer D. (1994) Safety in the andrology laboratory. In *Practical Laboratory Andrology*. Oxford Universtiy Press, New York, pp. 327–335.

Tsirigotis M., Hutchon S., Yazdani N. & Craft I. (1995) The value of oestradiol estimations in controlled ovarian hyperstimulation cycles (letter). *Human Reproduction* **10**, 972–973.

World Health Organization (1992) *WHO laboratory manual for the examination of human semen and sperm-cervical mucus interaction,* 3rd edition. Cambridge University Press, Cambridge.

# 3
# Patient selection and management

GODWIN I. MENIRU and FIDELIS T. AKAGBOSU

**Introduction**

About one in six couples existing in stable relationships will have some difficulty, at one time or the other, in achieving pregnancy. For the lucky ones this problem is only temporary and unaided conception eventually occurs after a variable length of time. For others, medical intervention is required, and the choice of a particular treatment depends on specific considerations, not least of which is the aetiology of the infertile condition. Intrauterine insemination (IUI) of prepared sperm suspension in a superovulated cycle fulfils criteria for classification as an assisted conception treatment. There is deliberate selection of a more fertile sperm population during laboratory preparation of semen samples. The prepared sperm suspension is deposited in the uterine cavity and, in some cases, even in the fallopian tubes. Multiple ovulation is induced and the ovulated oocytes come in contact with a high sperm density in the fallopian tubes.

The appeal of IUI lies in the fact that it is less invasive and cheaper to carry out than the more complex assisted conception treatments such as in vitro fertilisation (IVF) and embryo transfer, gamete intrafallopian transfer (GIFT), or their variants. The full benefits of IUI, however, may not be realised until details of factors that control outcome of treatment are clear. One such factor is patient selection as inappropriate application of this treatment to the whole of the infertile population will obscure its efficacy. Who then are suitable candidates for IUI? This is not an easy question to answer because although artificial insemination in general has been practised for more than 100 years, the current approach to IUI has only been in clinical use for a relatively short time. Furthermore, conflicting results have been reported in the recent literature making it difficult to identify groups of patients who will benefit maximally from this treatment. Some indications are largely empirical at present, but it is still possible to deduce a broad group of people in whom this treatment may be applicable.

Interestingly, GIFT shares many similarities with IUI as in both procedures gamete density is increased at the natural site of fertilisation in the fallopian tube, with the expectation that this will overcome defects in the innate reproductive potential of the couples involved. The major difference is that while the sperm concentration and number of oocytes replaced in the fallopian tube during GIFT are known, it is not certain how many ovulated oocytes are successfully picked up by the fallopian tubes in an IUI treatment cycle. Moreover, the presence, viability and concentration of sperm at the ampulla at the time of ovulation and tubal oocyte pickup cannot be documented. These notwithstanding, it is tempting to propose that generally similar indications should apply to both techniques in which case IUI will become a much preferred option by virtue of the fact that it is simpler, less invasive and cheaper. Provided an intelligent and compassionate approach to this matter is adopted it is not likely that patients will be treated inappropriately, especially when it is remembered that most of those who get pregnant with IUI usually do so within the first three to four cycles of treatment (Plosker *et al.* 1994; Comhaire 1995; Ombelet *et al.* 1995b; Campana *et al.* 1996). By corollary, those who do not succeed in getting pregnant within that time frame should be re-evaluated with a view to offering them IVF. This is the approach that will be adopted during the following account of indications for IUI.

It must be stated at this point that any couple being considered for IUI should have been evaluated by means of a thorough clinical history, physical examination, semen analysis, post-coital test, day 21 progesterone assay to confirm ovulatory cycles, a hysterosalpingogram and/or diagnostic laparoscopy combined with chromotubation. The reader should note that 'IUI' as described in this chapter entails superovulation, timed administration of an ovulatory dose of human chorionic gonadotrophin, semen preparation in the laboratory and injection of the sperm suspension into the uterine cavity.

**Insemination with fresh husband sperm**

*Male factors*

*Retrograde ejaculation*

A number of conditions may lead to reflux of semen backwards from the posterior urethra and into the bladder at the time of ejaculation. These include diabetes mellitus, multiple sclerosis, drugs such as alpha-adrenergic blockers and phenothiazines. Damage to the innervation of the bladder neck can occur during surgery, for example transurethral resection of the prostate and retropubic prostatectomy. Diagnosis is by the demonstration of sperm or the detection of fructose in the urine following an orgasm. These spermatozoa may be alive initially but rapidly lose their viability due to the toxic effects, hypotonicity and acidity of urine.

The goal of management is to alkalinise urine and retrieve the sperm as soon as possible after ejaculation. Mortimer (1994) described a protocol for this. Three days of abstinence from ejaculation are required and one tablespoonful of sodium bicarbonate dissolved in a cup of water is taken on the morning and night of the third day. A fresh solution of sodium bicarbonate is also drunk on the morning of the procedure. Prior to masturbation the bladder is emptied; urine is then passed into a sterile container as soon as possible following masturbation. Details of laboratory extraction of sperm from the urine sample can be found in Mortimer (1994). Basically, the urine sample is aliquoted immediately into tubes and centrifuged to recover the sperm which forms a pellet at the bottom of the tube. This pellet is then resuspended in culture medium and processed in a series of wash-centrifugation steps which may incorporate a bouyant density gradient medium and/or swim-up (see Chapter 8). The prepared sperm suspension is then used for IUI. Alternative regimens for alkalinising urine and controlling its osmolarity are described in Yavetz *et al.* (1994). A more invasive method entails emptying the bladder of all urine with a catheter and instilling a small quantity of embryo culture medium or any other physiological buffered solution into it. Following orgasm the bladder is emptied again with a catheter and the fluid prepared as described above to recover the sperm.

It is also possible for these men to have anterograde ejaculation as has been demonstrated by Crich & Jequier (1978) (J. Crich; personal communication) but this takes training and persistence. Essentially the patient is asked to try and ejaculate during masturbation or sexual intercourse with a full bladder. The reasoning behind this is that urinary continence with a full bladder entails closure of the bladder neck sphincters and this prevents reflux of ejaculated semen into the bladder, especially when the patient is in an upright position. Marmar *et al.* (1977) asked their patients to alkalinise their urine before intercourse and void into the vagina after an orgasm. This alternative to artificial insemination with recovered sperm does not seem to have been popular. Natural conception is however possible with these manoeuvres. Surgical treatments aimed at restoring sphincteric control to the bladder base were described by Abrahams *et al.* (1975), Ramadan *et al.* (1985) and Middleton & Urry (1986). Medical therapy is also possible and aims at either increasing sympathetic discharge or decreasing parasympathetic activity at the bladder neck (Yavetz *et al.* 1994). Alpha-adrenergic agents such as phenylpropanolamine hydrochloride, synephrine and nidodrin and anticholinergic drugs like brompheniramine, have been used quite successfully in this regard (Andalaro & Dube 1975; Budd 1975; Thiagarajah *et al.* 1978; Sandler 1979; Brooks *et al.* 1980; Schill 1990).

### *Impotence or ejaculatory dysfunction*

These may have organic or psychogenic causes. Psychological assessment and therapy are more appropriate primary treatment when the latter factors are culpable. Details of these are beyond the scope of this chapter and suitable texts should be consulted for further information on their use for the management of psychogenic impotence, ejaculatory failure and premature ejaculation. Organic causes include spinal cord injury, diabetes mellitus, multiple sclerosis, atherosclerosis, hypo- or hyperthyroidism, epilepsy and renal failure. Ejaculatory failure can occur as a result of damage to the hypogastric nerves during abdominal surgery such as abdominoperineal resection of the rectum, retroperitoneal lymph node dissection and aorto-iliac surgery (Doyle & Hirsh 1992). Drugs are also an important cause of these problems (Table 3.1). Initial efforts should be aimed at the treatment of these causal conditions but if sexual impairment is permanent, semen can be collected from these patients through other means (Table 3.2) (Rainsbury 1992). The penile vibrator or rectal electrostimulator are effective and relatively safe for the induction of emission of seminal fluid from these men. There is a slight risk of causing autonomic hypereflexia in men with spinal cord injury and this manifests with a rapidly rising blood pressure following orgasm. This makes it imperative for the procedures to be carried out only by a team of properly trained and experienced personnel and in suitably equipped operating theatre units. Some prophylactic measures and drug treatment are available for this complication (Rainsbury 1992). Care has to be exercised in the use of the probes to avoid causing rectal perforation and burns to the mucosa of the rectum. Retrograde ejaculation can also occur in such men, so the bladder is emptied and some amount of embryo culture medium instilled into it prior to the procedure. This is drained off and processed immediately after emission has taken place.

The quality of semen is generally poor in men who are continent for long periods such as the above group of patients. Although the sperm density might be increased in the ejaculate, the motility is low. Furthermore, debris, inflammatory cells and quite often bacteria, usually abound in the sample. These patients have recurrent urinary tract infection which ultimately spreads to affect the prostate, epididymides and testes, leading to blockage of

Table 3.1. *Drugs involved in the causation of impotence and ejaculatory dysfunction*

*Sedatives and antidepressants*
Amitryptiline
Chlordiazepoxide
Chlorpromazine
Diazepam
Imipramine
Monoamine oxidase inhibitors
Perphenazine
Phenelzine sulphate
Thioridazine
Trifluoperazine hydrochloride

*Antihypertensive agents*
Clonidine
Guanethidine sulphate
Hydralazine
Methyldopa
Metoprolol
Phenoxybenzamine hydrochloride
Prazosin hydrochloride
Propranolol
Reserpine
Spironolactone
Thiazide diuretics

*Drugs of abuse*
Alcohol
Cocaine
Codeine
Heroin
Nicotine
Methadone
Pethidine

*Others*
Clofibrate
Cimetidine
Digoxin
Ketoconazole

Table 3.2. *Methods of obtaining semen in irremediable impotence*

*Intracavernosal injections*
Papavarine hydrochloride
Phenoxybenzamine
Phentolamine mesylate
Prostaglandins

*Surgical methods*
Epididymal sperm aspiration
Hypogastric plexus stimulator
Sperm reservoirs

*Penile vibrator*

*Rectal electrostimulation*

glandular ducts as well as impairment of spermatogenesis. Direct effects on testicular function occur from chronic elevation of scrotal temperature in wheelchair-bound patients. Because of these problems it is clear that the assisted conception treatment to be offered depends on individual circumstances and semen quality. Rainsbury (1992) described a protocol which is based on the best three semen analysis results of each patient; patients are offered intravaginal insemination, IUI or in vitro fertilisation (IVF) depending on these results. As a general guide, conventional IVF or intracytoplasmic sperm injection (ICSI) should be carried out when the total motile count of recovered sperm is less than one million. IUI is offered when higher counts are obtained.

### Hypospadias

In cases of severe hypospadias, deposition of semen occurs either outside the vagina or at a distance from the cervical os such that the intervening acidic vaginal environment decimates the sperm before they reach the os. IUI is a logical solution to this problem and the first reported case of artificial insemination was actually in a patient with hypospadias. He was said to have been told by John Hunter to collect his ejaculate and inject it into his wife's vagina with a syringe. The modern approach to the finding of hypospadias at birth is however that of surgical repair during infancy or childhood. Hypospadias should therefore be a rare indication for IUI nowadays.

*Hypospermia*

The normal ejaculate volume is taken to be 2 ml and above (WHO 1992) and hypospermia is said to exist if the volume is less than this. This finding becomes more significant if it is constant in all semen samples collected by the patient. Although obvious, it still has to be confirmed that the low volume is not because of spillage of semen at the time of collection. As an adequate level of sexual excitement is required for optimal emission to occur, the patient may be asked to masturbate at home and bring in the sample for analysis rather than producing it on site. Congenital absence of the seminal vesicles or blockage of the ejaculatory ducts may be responsible for a low ejaculate volume but loss of part of the ejaculate through reflux into the bladder has to be excluded by examining a post-orgasmic urine sample for sperm after centrifugation, or for fructose. The importance of hypospermia lies in the fact that in severe cases the very small volume of ejaculate may be deposited well away from the cervix and the sperm do not come in contact with the external os. Furthermore, the small volume of seminal plasma is inadequate to raise the pH of the upper vagina and the sperm rapidly become overwhelmed by the vaginal acidity. IUI provides an easy means of treating this disorder as semen is collected, prepared in the laboratory and the resulting sperm suspension deposited in the uterine cavity thereby preventing their destruction in the vagina.

*Non-liquefying or highly viscous semen*

Semen rapidly coagulates after ejaculation but liquefaction usually commences within 5 minutes and is complete by 40–60 minutes if the sample is kept at room temperature, or sooner if incubated at 37 °C. The seminal vesicles produce enzymes that bring about coagulation of the semen while liquefaction is caused by seminine which is produced by the prostate gland. Complete or partial failure of liquefaction may be noted in some individuals but the usual finding is actually that of a sample that has liquefied but remains highly viscous. Theoretically this increased viscosity impedes the escape of sperm from the ejaculate into the cervical canal before destruction by vaginal acidity occurs; it is hard to document the contribution of this finding to the causation of infertility. Semen of increased viscosity may be produced by men who have fathered children. Besides, highly viscous ejaculates often have portions showing normal viscosity and sperm contained in this portion should be capable of gaining access to the cervical canal and upper parts of the female genital tract. Enzymatic digestion of the mucus is possible with plasmin or chymotrypsin (WHO 1992) but it is not clear how many centres use such techniques prior to analysis or preparation of viscous semen samples. Mechanical methods are usually employed to break the tenacious mucus threads at the outset of sperm preparation. An aliquot of culture medium is added to the semen sample followed by repeated aspiration and expulsion through a size 19G hypodermic needle. Alternatively, this mixture can be drawn in and out of a polystyrene serological pipette if the sample is not too viscous.

*Subnormal sperm parameters*

Semen analysis provides an indirect estimate of a man's fertility potential. The World Health Organization defines a normal semen sample as containing 20 million or more sperm per millilitre of ejaculate, with 50% or more of them showing forward progression and 30% or more having normal morphology (WHO 1992). This does not mean that men with lower values are incapable of fathering children but there is a general trend towards decreased fertility with a decline in these and other related parameters. The usefulness of IUI in couples with subnormal sperm parameters is still controversial. While many studies show good pregnancy rates in such cases others fail to find support for the use of IUI in these patients (references in Ombelet *et al.* 1995b). This non-agreement is not surprising given the myriad impediments to meaningful comparison of results from various studies on the efficacy of IUI (see Chapter 14).

The mechanism whereby subnormal sperm parameters decrease natural fertility probably depends on the particular abnormality. In oligozoospermia a decreased number of sperm is presented to the cervical os, consequently decreasing the number that will successfully negotiate the canal and reach the site of fertilisation in the fallopian tubes. A similar problem exists in situations of asthenozoospermia because there is a decrease in the proportion of motile sperm in the ejaculate and their progression may also be impaired. Even those that manage to reach the ampulla of the fallopian tube may not have the required motility characteristics required to break through the egg investments in order to reach and fertilise the egg. In patients with oligoasthenozoospermia the normal motile sperm fraction is selected out during the preparation of the semen sample and by being deposited in the uterine cavity sperms bypass the vaginal acidity and cervix, and reach the fallopian tubes in greater numbers than would have otherwise been possible. Infertility due to teratozoospermia arises in a slightly different way although the abnormal morphology could also interfere with the motility pattern of the sperm; binding of the sperm head to the zona pellucida prior to penetration is impossible in certain varieties of abnormal morphology that involve the sperm head. Sperm preparation and deposition in the uterine cavity are not likely to improve the chances of fertilisation in such cases except if an adequate number of normally formed motile sperm is selected out from the semen sample during preparation. This is more likely if the total motile sperm count in the ejaculate is high and teratozoospermia is not 100%.

Ombelet *et al.* (1995a) made some important observations in their study of 1100 consecutive IUI cycles. Of interest was the fact that they found similar pregnancy rates in couples with unexplained, female factor only or male factor infertility. Furthermore, men with subnormal semen parameters had similar pregnancy rates with those who had normal parameters, provided the prepared sperm suspension contained more than 300 000 motile sperm with at least 10% of them showing Grade 'A' progression (WHO 1992). An even higher pregnancy rate was obtained when the sperm density exceeded 1 000 000 in the inseminated sample. In a recent report, Campana *et al.* (1996) confirmed that pregnancies were still possible when less than 500 000 sperm were inseminated but they also showed significant improvement of pregnancy rates when this count exceeded 1 000 000. A multicentre trial comparing ovulation induction alone or in combination with intraperitoneal insemination (IPI), IUI, IVF and GIFT has substantiated the efficacy of IUI in the management of infertility due to subnormal semen parameters (Crosignani & Walters 1994). In that report IUI, GIFT and IVF had a mean pregnancy rate per cycle of 21.2% while that of IPI and ovulation induction was 6.8%. It appears that the minimum prepared sperm count required for successful IUI is similar to that of IVF (Comhaire *et al.* 1995).

### Female factors

#### Vaginismus

This has been a traditional indication for intravaginal insemination but it is not appropriate for artificial insemination to be carried out in this group of women unless there have been persistent failures at psychological intervention and the couple have strong wishes for pregnancy. IUI may not be easy here because transvaginal ultrasound scanning will be needed for monitoring of the patient's response to superovulation. Furthermore, insertion of a vaginal speculum to enable visualisation and cannulation of the cervix may not be possible unless it is carried out under general anaesthesia. Finally, obstetrical management following successful establishment of pregnancy has to be discussed including the fact that vaginal examinations may be necessary at some stage during pregnancy. The planned route of delivery has to be discussed and agreed upon. Epidural analgesia is certainly indicated for this group of women during labour.

Table 3.3 *Fertility-related functions of the cervix and its mucus*

Control of sperm entry into the upper genital tract
Protection of sperm from vaginal acidity and phagocytosis
Nutrition of sperm
Selection of sperm based on motility characteristics
Sperm reservoir function
Initiation of capacitation

*Cervical factor*

Cervical mucus is produced by secretory cells of the endocervix but the endometrium and lining of the fallopian tubes also contribute to this fluid. It is also possible that some amount of fluid from the peritoneal cavity and ruptured ovarian follicles pass through the fallopian tubes to reach the uterine cavity and eventually the cervical canal. More than 90% of cervical mucus is made up of water while mucin, white blood cells and cellular debris, such as endometrial and cervical cells, make up the rest. Oestradiol stimulates the production of a copious watery mucus whose volume reaches 500 μl/day at midcycle while progesterone inhibits the production of mucus by the endocervical cells. The main functions of the cervix in relation to conception are shown on Table 3.3. Optimal conditions for entry and migration of sperm through the cervical canal are present at midcycle, just before ovulation occurs. Interaction between spermatozoa and cervical mucus can be assessed in vivo with the post-coital test and in vitro with the slide and sperm-cervical-mucus-contact tests (WHO 1992; Moghissi 1993).

It is a well known fact that the cervical factor (Table 3.4) is not well assessed during investigation of infertile couples despite being involved in 5–10% of cases (Moghissi 1993). Evaluation of midcycle cervical mucus, which may yield important information, is not commonly carried out. Furthermore, the clinical value of tests such as the post-coital test is controversial and this is probably due to the lack of standardisation of the scoring system, timing of the tests and interpretation of results. A negative test result may indicate the presence of a cervical factor but it may also be due to the lack of coitus, ejaculation, intra-vaginal ejaculation or incorrect timing of the test in relation to the menstrual cycle or sexual intercourse. The existence of a cervical factor can also be suspected from the clinical history and findings on vaginal examination but the presence of characteristic preovulatory mucus largely diminishes the importance of a clinical history of cervical surgery (Table 3.4). Cervical stenosis is more likely to cause infertility if it arises in association with a previous oper-

Table 3.4. *Cervical causes of infertility*

---

*Inspissated cervical mucus (e.g. cystic fibrosis)*

*Deficient or absent cervical mucus production*
cone biopsy
cervical amputation
radical cauterisation, diathermy or cryotherapy of the cervical canal
colpoperineorrhaphy
deep long loop excision of the transformation zone

*Tumour of endocervix (leiomyoma or polyp)*

*Severe cervical stenosis*

*Hostile cervical mucus*

*Chronic endocervicitis*

---

ative procedure that caused significant damage to the endocervical secretory cells. Cervical mucus hostility is said to be present if the mucus is acidic, has increased viscosity or cellularity, or contains antisperm antibodies.

IUI in patients with cervical factor infertility is generally effective because it bypasses the cervical block to sperm entry into the upper genital tract (Glezerman 1993; Martinez *et al.* 1993). Pregnancy rates of between 52 and 70% have been reported in the literature (Barwin 1974; White & Glass 1976; Glezerman *et al.* 1984; Sher *et al.* 1984; Wiltbank *et al.* 1985).

*Ovulatory dysfunction*

A broad range of problems cause ovulatory dysfunction which accounts for 30–40% of female factor infertility. Details of these disorders may be found in relevant texts (Breckwoldt *et al.* 1993; Rowe *et al.* 1993). Treatment depends on the particular problem but some cases may require ovulation induction which, if combined with timed sexual intercourse, can result in pregnancy. The problem is how long to persist with this management in the face of continued failure to conceive despite documented ovulation and the absence of an obvious impediment to the ascent of sperm up the female genital tract. If assisted conception treatment is eventually offered, should IUI be the first option rather than IVF? The study by Plosker *et al.* (1994) shows quite clearly that IUI is an effective treatment for these couples. They found a pregnancy rate of 45.8% per patient and 30% per cycle following IUI in couples where the female partner had ovulatory dysfunction and failed treatment following ovulation induction and timed sexual intercourse. This rate was, in fact, significantly greater than those found in couples with other causes of infertility in that study.

### Allergy to semen

The use of IUI for the management of allergy to seminal fluid was reported by Shapiro *et al.* (1981). The nulligravid patient had presented some years previously with a history of increasingly severe attacks of urticaria and laryngeal oedema each time she had sexual intercourse. Extensive immunological evaluation confirmed the allergen to be seminal fluid proteins and the use of condoms was advised to prevent further contact with semen. IUI was subsequently carried out in seven natural cycles before she became pregnant and later delivered twin babies. In each cycle of treatment, sperm preparation involved two wash steps with culture medium, layering over albumin columns and then another wash step. This preparation method was effective in eliminating all allergens from the sample. This is obviously a rare indication for IUI.

### Poor follicular response to superovulation for IVF

There are occasions during superovulation for IVF treatment when a patient responds suboptimally with development of ovarian follicles whose number does not justify exposing the patient to the potential dangers and cost of oocyte retrieval and IVF. The main options here are to abandon the treatment cycle completely, ask the couple to have intercourse following administration of an ovulatory dose of human chorionic gonadotrophin injection, or to convert to an IUI cycle, provided there is no documented tubal pathology. Evidence in support of the latter option is sparse and there may be a fear that this constitutes an abuse of IUI and will jeopardise results. Ombelet *et al.* (1995a) however achieved a pregnancy rate of 10.9% (11 pregnancies in 101 cancelled IVF cycles) for this unusual indication for IUI. It is of interest to note that this pregnancy rate was not significantly different from that of 13.8% obtained in a group of patients who had planned IUI in the same unit.

### Endometriosis

This is a relatively common gynaecological problem, being present in 10–25% of females with gynaecological complaints in the western world. It is still an enigma in many ways, one of which is in its relationship to infertility. While the effect of moderate to severe disease (American Fertility Society 1985) on fertility is more obvious, the link with asymptomatic mild to minimal disease is tenuous and hence controversial. If such a connection exists, possible mechanisms will include defective ovarian, tubal, endometrial, sperm and coital function, and recurrent early pregnancy failure caused by chemical agents released by endometriotic tissue and other reactive phenomena such as macrophage invasion and phagocytosis of sperm (Shaw 1992). The fact that endometriosis is seen more commonly in infertile females than in fertile controls (Shaw 1992) lends further support to a causal role but additional evidence is required before the exact relationship can be determined with any degree of certainty. The lack of unanimity also extends to the issue of treatment for mild endometriosis in infertile women but it is safe to say that expectant management should be carried out in asymptomatic patients. Medical and/or surgical treatment of moderate and severe disease may be aimed at the control of symptoms or treatment of infertility. Symptoms tend to recur following cessation of treatment and medical treatment prolongs the infertile situation because ovarian/menstrual function is often abolished for periods of 6 months and upwards. Moreover, restoration of normal fertility is not invariable following these treatments and many patients will eventually require assisted conception treatment. IVF or GIFT is effective treatment for infertility in these women when carried out with a drug protocol that includes the use of gonadotrophin releasing hormone agonists (Edwards & Brody 1995). IUI is also an option if the ovaries are free of disease (Edwards & Brody 1995) but reported pregnancy rates vary widely. A mean pregnancy rate of 11.5% (range 0–18%) was found by Martinez *et al.* (1993) in their review of seven studies. A retrospective study on the use of IUI for the management of various aetiologies of infertility revealed a cycle pregnancy rate of 8% for patients with endometriosis, which was significantly lower than the rates obtained for couples with ovulatory dysfunction (30%), male factor (14%) and unexplained infertility (13%) (Plosker *et al.* 1994).

### *Factors common to both male and female*

#### *Immunological infertility*

Antisperm antibodies may be found in a variety of body compartments (Table 3.5) and available evidence suggests that there is an increased incidence of this problem in infertile couples (Bronson *et al.* 1984; Marshburn & Kutteh 1994). Locally elaborated antisperm antibodies are more important in the causation of infertility than those found in the serum. Broadly speaking these antibodies either impair sperm movement up the female genital tract or prevent binding of the sperm to the zona pellucida preparatory to fertilisation. Formation of antisperm antibodies in men tends to occur in situations of obstruction or trauma to the male genital tract such as congenital obstruction of the vas deferens, following vasectomy and multiple testicular biopsies. Receptive anal intercourse has been associated with the presence of antisperm antibodies in serum

Table 3.5. *Where antisperm antibodies can be found*

| Males | Females |
|---|---|
| Serum | Serum |
| Seminal fluid | Cervical mucus |
| | Tubal fluid |
| | Follicular fluid |
| | Peritoneal fluid |

(Marshburn & Kutteh 1994). Sperm antigen inoculation through a break in the continuity of the vaginal epithelium, theoretically at least, may explain the development of antisperm antibodies by some women. Other possible routes of inoculation include peritoneal instillation, receptive anal and oral intercourse.

Antisperm antibodies are a relative rather than an absolute cause of infertility and other causes of infertility, which may coexist in the same couple, have to be excluded or identified by systematic evaluation using well-established protocols. This is particularly important because results of clinical treatment of immunological infertility have not been very encouraging. Prolonged use of condoms (for 6–9 months) has been proposed as a means of preventing further contact of semen with the female genital tract in women who are already sensitised, with the hope that this will lead to a fall in the serum antisperm antibody level. There is no evidence that this works as it has not led to increased pregnancy rates following discontinuation of condom use (Kremer 1979). Immunosuppression with steroids appears to be effective in some studies while in others no benefit on the conception rate has been noticed (Marshburn & Kutteh 1994). This treatment modality has not been widely employed by fertility workers most probably due to well-known effects of prolonged usage of steroids at high doses. Laboratory procedures aimed at removing antisperm antibodies from the surface of spermatozoa are not very successful and some decrease the viability of the sperm even further.

ICSI has been shown to have the best success rate of all assisted conception treatment modalities in this group of infertile patients and should be carried out in severe cases. IUI still has a role here and a diagnostic conventional IVF treatment cycle may be necessary before committing patients to ICSI. IUI is ideally carried out in couples with antisperm antibodies in the cervical mucus. The cervix is bypassed and sperm is deposited higher up in the female genital tract, although sperm that subsequently gravitate to the cervical canal may become immobilised by antibodies in the mucus. There is however a chance that such women may have these antibodies also in the secretions of the upper genital tract and these will immobilise sperm deposited there by IUI. Even though some types of sperm-bound antisperm antibodies of seminal fluid origin will not impede the ascent of sperm up the female genital tract, they may interfere with subsequent interactions between the sperm and oocyte. All these notwithstanding it is probably worth trying a few cycles of IUI in properly selected cases of immunological infertility.

## Unexplained infertility

Standard investigations (Van den Eede 1995) fail to reveal a cause for the infertile condition in about 10–25% of couples (Crosignani *et al.* 1991; Edwards and Brody 1995) and they are said to have idiopathic or unexplained infertility. More extensive evaluation, however, decreases the incidence of this diagnosis. Some identified pathologies may also be found in a significant proportion of fertile couples thereby making it more difficult to ascertain their true relevance (Crosignani *et al.* 1993). Issues become more complicated when these infertile couples become pregnant despite their earlier diagnosis. Irrespective of the absence of a diagnosed cause, there comes a time when a decision has to be taken regarding the need for assisted conception treatment especially in cases of prolonged infertility or increasing age of the female partner (Jansen 1995). At such times, terminology like 'treatment-independent pregnancy rates' become irrelevant because medical intervention is actively sought for the speedy resolution of the state of infertility, rather than continuing with watchful expectancy. IUI definitely has a role here because it incorporates interventions that could overcome subtle unrecognised fertility defects in these couples. A multicentre trial on the efficacy of superovulation alone or in combination with IPI, IUI, IVF and GIFT for the management of unexplained infertility provides support for this proposal (Crosignani *et al.* 1991). In that study superovulation in combination with IPI, IUI, IVF or GIFT achieved a pregnancy rate of about 27% per cycle which was significantly greater than the rate of 15.2% for superovulation alone and the calculated treatment-independent spontaneous pregnancy rate of 1.11%. IUI is the least invasive of the above effective options. A review of published reports (Martinez *et al.* 1993) has confirmed the efficacy of IUI in patients with unexplained infertility.

## Insemination with frozen husband sperm

### Absentee husband

Some occupations involve separation of couples for a significant part of their early lives together. One partner may travel away from home for relatively long periods of time or work in shifts that do not correspond with the other partner's work schedule. These limit opportunities for sexual intercourse to take place at optimal periods of the menstrual cycle and worsen any pre-existing mild subfertility to the extent that the couple find it difficult achieving pregnancy during the same time frame as other couples who are not encumbered by similar occupational impediments.

Imprisonment of the male partner of a couple may adversely affect their reproductive aspirations and many such couples do not have any moral, social or legal impediment to their continued procreation. Couples often travel for long distances to other cities or countries for assisted conception treatment such as IUI and IVF. Economic reasons often necessitate the husband's early return home while the wife remains behind to await scheduled treatments or repeat treatment cycles. All these couples could benefit from IUI using cryopreserved husband semen. Exclusion of those with subnormal semen parameters will improve the efficacy of treatment.

### Anti-neoplastic treatment

Therapy for malignancies tends to jeopardise subsequent reproductive function and many oncologists would advise cryostorage of several semen samples prior to commencement of chemotherapy, and radiotherapy if the testes are to be irradiated. Semen is also stored prior to orchiectomy for testicular tumours and an increasing number of males avail themselves of this opportunity to safeguard their potential for biological parentage. Following completion of their treatment, IUI can be carried out with the thawed prepared semen sample. Extensive pre-storage counselling is required to make sure the patient understands the implications, especially as they relate to his altered life expectancy. Comprehensive patient information should be provided and signed consents obtained. These consents should in addition to other facts, address the fate of stored semen in the event of the patient dying before their utilisation. The patient should also understand that success at assisted conception treatment with his stored semen is not guaranteed. This becomes more important in those cases of poor semen quality prior to cryopreservation; the advent of ICSI has however improved the outlook for these males.

### Vasectomy

The predicted boom in cryobanking of semen as a form of insurance prior to vasectomy does not seem to have materialised. Anyone contemplating this step should produce many samples of semen for cryopreservation and post-thaw analysis for sperm survival should be carried out before the vasectomy. It is not likely that this will become a major indication for IUI with frozen husband semen.

### Poor semen parameters

Theoretically, it is possible to cryopreserve several poor quality semen samples and pool them together later on for preparation and IUI. Unfortunately such samples will also have poor survival rates following thawing, making this an inefficient method of managing infertility caused by subnormal semen. Aboulghar *et al.* (1991) developed a slightly different approach and reported their study of two groups of patients, both with oligoasthenozoospermia. One group (Group A) had IUI using fresh husband sperm while IUI was deferred in the second group (Group B). Regular semen analysis was carried out every 2–4 weeks, for up to 8 months, to detect episodic improvement in the semen quality. Semen samples of improved quality were frozen and subsequently thawed for preparation and IUI. Prior to insemination the prepared thawed sperm sample was combined with another sperm suspension prepared from a fresh ejaculate that was produced on that day. Analysis of data from Group A showed a pregnancy rate per cycle of 4.1% and a cumulative rate per patient, after three cycles, of 13%. Corresponding rates for Group B were 9.1% and 27.7%; this difference was statistically significant. Further examination of Group B showed that those in whom the objective of freezing improved semen samples was achieved (Group B1) had even higher rates of 12.3% per cycle and 36% after three cycles while those in whom the poor quality semen profile remained unchanged during the period of monitoring (Group B2) had lower rates of 5.8% and 17.7%, respectively. The poor quality semen samples collected by patients in Group B2 had been frozen and prepared in exactly the same way as improved samples produced by patients in Group B1. There was no significant difference between the pregnancy rates of Groups A and B2. This protocol certainly merits further study and emulation if these results are confirmed. It will also be interesting to find out what effect, if any, addition of the prepared fresh sample to the inseminate had on pregnancy rates.

### Other drug therapy

There is an increasing awareness of drugs that have detrimental effects on testicular function (Table 3.6) (Forman *et al.* 1996). Some are drugs of abuse while others are medications used for the treatment of various ailments. The effect of these drugs may be permanent or reversible following discontinuation of their ingestion and the degree of deterioration in semen quality varies from mild abnormalities in semen parameters to azoospermia. The correct management is for discontinuation of the drug in question but this may not be easy in addicts who need an established care and support system to help them achieve that objective. Medications like sulphasalazine and niridazole have less damaging

Table 3.6. *Drugs that exert detrimental effects on testicular function*

*Known toxins*
Alcohol
Cocaine
Colchicine
Diethylstilboestrol (maternal administration)
Methadone
Heroin
Lead
Niridazole
Sulphasalazine
Tobacco
Trinitrotoluene

*Suspected toxins*
Amantadine
Antiepileptics
Calcium channel blockers (verapamil and nifedipine)
Propranolol

*Source:* Compiled from Forman *et al.* (1996)

alternatives which could be substituted for use by patients. There may however be situations where alternatives are not suitable for a particular patient, in which case semen samples are frozen before commencing treatment and used later on for IUI or IVF if required.

**Insemination with donor sperm**

Insemination with donor sperm can be carried out for a number of reasons (Table 3.7) but the main indications relate to male factor infertility. In previous years use of donor sperm was the only realistic way couples with irremediable azoospermia or severely subnormal semen parameters could have children. IUI was carried out with thawed frozen semen. With the advent of ICSI and other microassisted fertilisation techniques, many of these men are now able to become genetic parents with their own sperm because only a few viable sperms are required for ICSI of all collected oocytes. Some couples may still require donor insemination especially those who have had multiple failures at IVF/ICSI with an attendant toll on their finances and other aspects of their life.

Transmission of serious hereditary diseases can be prevented by the use of

Table 3.7. *Indications for donor insemination*

Azoospermia of primary testicular origin
Severely subnormal semen parameters
Persistent failure at IVF/ICSI
Hereditary disease
Rhesus isoimmunisation
Single woman
Lesbian couple

*Notes:*
ICSI: intracytoplasmic sperm injection; IVF: in vitro fertilisation.

donor semen. Another option for affected couples would be for IVF to be carried out and pre-implantation embryo biopsy and cytogenetic studies performed on the embryos generated by the procedure. Embryos that are eventually transferred back into the uterine cavity would be from the group that do not carry genetic markers of the disease being investigated.

Maternal Rhesus isoimmunisation is now uncommon due to well-established screening programmes and prophylactic administration of Rhesus anti-D gamma globulin. Donor insemination may be the last hope for a couple where the woman has been sensitised and is unable to carry a Rhesus positive foetus to viability despite medical intervention. Before this is embarked upon, the other option of gestational surrogacy should be explored with the couple. The technology for IVF with the couple's gametes and transfer into a Rhesus positive gestational surrogate is already available and being used for other indications.

With relaxation of societal norms increasing numbers of single women and lesbian couples are now requesting the use of donor sperm for IUI. It will be interesting to find out if practitioners consider establishing tubal patency in these women before proceeding to IUI. Peculiar requirements in this group of patients will become clearer with time. A recent report highlighted one such need. It was found that a large proportion of lesbian couples who had donor insemination would prefer a female practitioner to perform the insemination rather than a male (Wendland *et al.* 1996).

### Conclusion

There is no doubt that IUI is an effective assisted conception treatment method but further experience will allow delineation of indicated patient groups so as

Table 3.8. *Contraindications to intrauterine insemination*

| |
|---|
| Tubal pathology |
| Genital tract infection |
| Severe semen abnormality |
| Genetic abnormality in husband |
| Unexplained genital tract bleeding |
| Pelvic mass |
| Older woman |
| Multiple infertility aetiologies |
| Pelvic surgery |
| Pregnancy contraindicated |
| Severe illness in one or both partners |
| Recent chemotherapy or radiotherapy |
| Multiple failures at IUI |

*Notes:*
IUI: intrauterine insemination.

to maximise the potentials of the treatment. At the same time it is very important to identify those in whom it is contraindicated either for medical reasons or because of the presence of poor prognostic factors (Table 3.8). Bilateral tubal blockage is an obvious contraindication but some workers will carry out IUI in patients with only one patent tube. This is one of the areas that has to be studied carefully because patency in such cases does not mean that tubal function is normal, especially if the other tube became blocked following an infection or was excised because of sequelae such as ectopic pregnancy. Increasing female age is associated with deterioration of natural fertility and a diminished response to assisted conception treatment and this operates mainly by way of decreasing oocyte quality. Plosker *et al.* (1994) found the pregnancy rate per cycle of IUI to be 4% in women above 40 years of age and 14% in those between 25 and 39 years. It is therefore important that older women presenting with infertility are treated with the best available modality which also provides practitioners with the opportunity to extract maximal information on indices such as oocyte quality, fertilisation and cleavage rates, and embryo quality. IVF fulfils these criteria and should be offered to such patients instead of IUI, although this does not mean that they cannot become pregnant through the latter procedure. The same situation holds for cases where multiple aetiologies for the infertile condition are detected as these have additive effects (Jansen 1995). Another guiding statistic is that most pregnancies achieved through IUI occur within the first three to four cycles of treatment. These number of cycles can be completed in less than a year, leaving ample time for other modalities such as conventional IVF or ICSI to be explored. It is also not mandatory to go through four cycles of IUI. Every failed cycle of treatment should be reviewed and information that will influence subsequent management of the patient's infertility extracted. The place of GIFT in patients who fail to conceive through IUI has not been resolved. This is because the reason for the failure may be rooted in events that take place behind sight in the fallopian tubes. GIFT will not provide any information on fertilisation and cleavage (Edwards & Brody 1995). It is better in such cases to carry out a 'diagnostic' IVF cycle. If fertilisation and cleavage are observed to be satisfactory GIFT can be offered, in subsequent cycles, to those who fail to become pregnant in that initial IVF cycle. Finally, this account has assumed that all practitioners involve their patients in the decision making process after providing them with clear unambiguous information on matters related to their reproductive welfare.

**References**

Aboulghar M. A., Mansour R. T., Serour G. I., Sattar M. A. & Elatter I. (1991) Cryopreservation of the ocassionally improved semen samples for intrauterine insemination: a new approach in the treatment of idiopathic male infertility. *Fertility and Sterility* **56,** 1151–1155.

Abrahams J., Solish G. I., Boorjian P. & Waterhouse R. K. (1975) The surgical correction of retrograde ejaculation. *Journal of Urology* **114,** 888–891.

Andaloro V. A. Jr & Dube A. (1975) Treatment of retrograde ejaculation with brompheniramine. *Urology* **5,** 520–522.

American Fertility Society. (1985) Revised American Fertility Society Classification of Endometriosis 1985. *Fertility and Sterility* **43,** 351–352.

Barwin B. N. (1974) Intrauterine insemination of husband's semen. *Journal of Reproduction and Fertility* **36,** 101–106.

Breckwoldt M., Zahradnik H. P. & Neulen J. (1993) Classification and diagnosis of ovarian insufficiency. In: *Infertility: Male and Female*. (V. Insler, B. Lunenfeld, eds), 2nd edition, Churchill Livingstone, Edinburgh, pp. 229–251.

Bronson R., Cooper G. & Rosenfield D. (1984) Sperm antibodies: their role in infertility. *Fertility and Sterility* **42,** 171–183.

Brooks M. E., Berezin M. & Braf Z. (1980) Treatment of retrograde ejaculation with imipramine. *Urology* **15,** 353–355.

Budd H. A. Jr (1975) Brompheniramine in treatment of retrograde ejaculation. (letter). *Urology* **6,** 131.

Campana A., Sakkas D., Stalberg A., Bianchi P. G., Comte I., Pache T. & Walker D. (1996) Intrauterine insemination: evaluation of the results according to the woman's age, sperm quality, total sperm count per insemination and life table analysis. *Human Reproduction* **11,** 732–736.

Comhaire F. (1995) Economic strategies in modern male subfertility treatment. *Human Reproduction*, **10** (supplement 1), 103–106.

Comhaire F., Milingos S., Liapi A., Gordts S., Campo R., Depypere H., Dhont M. & Schoonjans F. (1995) The effective cumulative pregnancy rate of different modes of treatment of male infertility. *Andrologia* **27,** 217–221.

Crich J. P. & Jequier A. M. (1978) Infertility in men with retrograde ejaculation: the action of urine on sperm motility and a simple method for achieving antegrade ejaculation. *Fertility and Sterility* **30**, 572–576.

Crosignani P. G., Collins J., Cooke I. D., Diczfalusy E. & Rubin B. (1993) Unexplained infertility. *Human Reproduction* **8**, 977–980.

Crosignani P. G. & Walters D. E. (1994) Clinical pregnancy and male subfertility; the ESHRE multicentre trial on the treatment of male subfertility. *Human Reproduction* **9**, 1112–1118.

Crosignani P. G., Walters D. E. & Soliani A. (1991) The ESHRE multicentre trial on the treatment of unexplained infertility: a preliminary report. *Human Reproduction* **6**, 953–958.

Doyle P. T. & Hirsh A. (1992) The investigation and treatment of infertile men. In: *A Textbook of In Vitro Fertilization and Assisted Reproduction*. (P. R. Brinsden, P. A. Rainsbury, eds.), The Parthenon Publishing Group, Carnforth, pp. 39–72.

Edwards R. G. & Brody S. A. (1995) Implantation rates during IVF, GIFT and other forms of assisted conception. In: *Principles and Practice of Assisted Human Reproduction*. W. B. Saunders Company, Philadelphia, pp. 475–518.

Forman R., Gilmour-White S. & Forman N. (1996) *Drug Induced Infertility and Sexual Dysfunction*. Cambridge University Press, Cambridge.

Glezerman M. (1993) Artificial insemination. In: *Infertility: Male and Female*. (V. Insler, B. Lunenfeld, eds), 2nd edition, Churchill Livingstone, Edinburgh, pp. 643–658.

Glezerman M., Bernstein D. & Insler V. (1984) The cervical factor of infertility and intrauterine insemination. *International Journal of Fertility* **29**, 16–19.

Jansen R. P. S. (1995) Elusive fertility: fecundability and assisted conception in perspective. *Fertility and Sterility* **64**, 252–254.

Kremer J. [1979] A new technique for intrauterine insemination. *International Journal of Fertility* **24**, 53–56.

Marmar J. L., Praiss D. E. & Debenedictis T. J. (1977) Postcoital voiding insemination. Technique for patients with retrograde ejaculation and infertility. *Urology* **9**, 288–290.

Marshburn P. B. & Kutteh W. H. (1994) The role of antisperm antibodies in infertility. *Fertility and Sterility* **61**, 799–811.

Martinez A. R., Bernardus R. E., Vermeiden J. P. W. & Schoemaker J. (1993) Basic questions on intrauterine insemination: an update. *Obstetrical and Gynecological Survey* **48**, 811–828.

Middleton R. J. & Urry R. L. (1986) The Young-Dees operation for the correction of retrograde ejaculation. *Journal of Urology* **136**, 1208–1209.

Moghissi K. S. (1993) Diagnosis and classification of disturbed sperm-cervical mucus interaction. In: *Infertility: Male and Female*. (V. Insler, B. Lunenfeld, eds), 2nd edition, Churchill Livingstone, Edinburgh, pp. 335–351.

Mortimer D. (1994) Therapeutic insemination procedures. In: *Practical Laboratory Andrology*. Oxford Universtiy Press, New York, pp. 287–299.

Ombelet W., Cox A., Jansen M., Vandeput H. & Bosmans E. (1995a) Artificial insemination (AIH). Artificial insemination 2: using the husband's sperm. In: *Diagnosis and Therapy of Male Factor in Assisted Reproduction*. (A. A. Acosta, T. F. Kruger, eds), The Parthenon Publishing Group, Carnforth, pp. 397–410.

Ombelet W., Puttemans P. & Bosmans E. (1995b) Intrauterine insemination: a first-step procedure in the algorithm of male subfertility treatment. *Human Reproduction* **10** (supplement), 90–102.

Plosker S. M., Jacobson W. & Amato P. (1994) Predicting and optimizing success in an intra-uterine insemination programme. *Human Reproduction* **9,** 2014–2021.

Rainsbury P. A. (1992) The treatment of male factor infertility due to sexual dysfunction. In: *A Textbook of In Vitro Fertilization and Assisted Reproduction.* (P. R. Brinsden, P. A. Rainsbury, eds), The Parthenon Publishing Group, Carnforth, pp. 345–359.

Ramadan A. E., El-Demiry M. I. M. & Ramadan A. E. (1985) Surgical correction of post-operative retrograde ejaculation. *British Journal of Urology* **57,** 458–461.

Rowe P. J., Comhaire F. H., Hargreave T. B. & Mellows H. J. (1993) *WHO Manual for the Standardized Investigation and Diagnosis of the Infertile Couple.* Cambridge University Press, Cambridge.

Sandler B. (1979) Idiopathic retrograde ejaculation. *Fertility and Sterility* **32,** 474–475.

Schill W. B. (1990) Pregnancy after brompheniramine treatment of a diabetic with incomplete emission failure. *Archives of Andrology* **25,** 101–104.

Shapiro S. S., Kooistra J. B., Schwartz D., Yunginger J. W. & Haning R. W. (1981) Induction of pregnancy in a woman with seminal plasma allergy. *Fertility and Sterility* **36,** 405–407.

Shaw R. W. (1992) Endometriosis. In: *Gynaecology.* (R. W. Shaw, W. P. Soutter, S. L. Stanton, eds), Churchill Livingstone, Edinburgh, pp. 421–435.

Sher G., Knutzen V. K., Stratton C. J., Montakhab M. M. & Allenson S. G. (1984) In vitro sperm capacitation and transcervical intrauterine insemination for the treatment of refractory infertility: Phase I. *Fertility and Sterility* **41,** 260–264.

Thiagarajah S., Darracott Vaughan E. Jr, Kitchin J. D., 3 (1978) Retrograde ejaculation: successful pregnancy following combined sympathomimetic medication and insemination. *Fertility and Sterility* **30,** 96–97.

Van den Eede B. (1995) Investigation and treatment of infertile couples: ESHRE guidelines for good clinical and laboratory practice. *Human Reproduction* **10,** 1246–1271.

Wendland C. L., Byrn F. & Hill C. (1996) Donor insemination: a comparison of lesbian couples, heterosexual couples and single women. *Fertility and Sterility* **65,** 764–770.

White R. M. & Glass R. H. (1976) Intrauterine insemination with husband's semen. *Obstetrics and Gynecology* **47,** 119–121.

Wiltbank M. C., Kosasa T. S. & Rogers B. J. (1985) Treatment of infertile patients by intrauterine insemination of washed spermatozoa. *Andrologia* **17,** 22–30.

World Health Organization (1992) *WHO laboratory manual for the examination of human semen and sperm-cervical mucus interaction,* third edition. Cambridge University Press, Cambridge.

Yavetz H., Yogev L., Hauser R., Lessing J. B., Paz G. & Homonnai Z. T. (1994) Retrograde ejaculation. *Human Reproduction* **9,** 381–386.

# 4
# Fertility counselling

ARLENE R. RAEBURN and MARYANN O. MENIRU

**Introduction**

The assisted reproduction technologies increasingly present fertility workers and their patients with innovative treatment methods. The success rates of the treatments are such that the chance of failure is on the average still higher than that of success in each cycle of treatment. It is in this climate of uncertainty, stress, disappointed expectations, continuing hope and emotional upheaval that fertility counselling has emerged as a distinct specialism of counselling. Fertility counselling can be described as the process of assisting individuals or couples to make informed decisions about their bioreproductive state. It covers apparently disparate areas such as infertility, pregnancy, miscarriage, termination of pregnancy, ectopic pregnancy and family planning. Clients can therefore be fertile, subfertile or infertile.

Previously, counselling in fertility treatment was felt to be appropriately carried out by clinicians and nurses but nowadays it is generally accepted that counselling is separate from the treatment roles, but complementary to them. The treatment team will frequently have to use counselling skills while they are in the process of treating patients. Furthermore, the nursing team are constantly called on to offer emotional support and a sympathetic listening ear to anxious patients. During consultations clinicians will need to give clear information and allow time for each couple to discuss the implications of each stage of treatment for them personally.

For many people going through fertility treatment the level of distress and tension can be greater than they expect. Treatment can also arouse very strong feelings related to incidents in the past, within present relationships, and may involve fear of the future. The role of the counsellor is essential in helping people to cope in some way with these crises which may be deeply affecting their lives. The Human Fertilisation and Embryology Authority (HFEA) has made a clear statement on the need for counselling and defined the three levels of counselling which they designate as essential. These are implications counselling, support counselling and therapeutic counselling (HFEA 1990). All members of the unit may offer the first two but the role of the counsellor encompasses implications, support and most importantly, therapeutic counselling. This chapter will discuss the role of the counsellor within the unit, the need for counselling at different stages of treatment, and also includes some clarification about the training and professional status of the counsellor.

### What is counselling?

Counselling is a word which many people use in diverse situations to describe the relationship between themselves and another person. Firstly it may be easier to define what it is not. It is not guidance, advice giving, befriending, caring in a parental way, 'treating' or 'healing' someone, instructing or teaching or using counselling skills in a helpful way (Sanders 1994). Counselling is an interpersonal way of working practised by a person, designated as counsellor, who is appropriately trained and who works by a recognised code of ethics and practice. Counselling only exists when the counsellor works respectfully with the client, and the client has agreed to be in a confidential counselling situation. The client must also feel safe and valued and experience the counsellor as non-judgemental in her approach. Through working in this way the client may gain a greater understanding of his or her life position and a sense of well-being may grow over time.

Further insights into the nature of counselling can be found in the Code of Ethics and Practice of the British Association of Counselling (BAC 1985). 'The overall aim of counselling is to provide an opportunity for the client to work towards living in a more satisfying and resourceful way. The term "counselling" includes work with individuals, pairs or groups of people, often but not always, referred to as "clients". The objectives of particular counselling relationships will vary according to the client's needs. Counselling may be concerned with developmental issues, addressing and resolving specific problems, making decisions, coping with crisis, developing personal insight and knowledge, working through feelings of inner conflict or improving relationships with others. The counsellor's role is to facilitate the client's work in ways which respect the client's values, personal resources and capacity for self-determination'. Counselling skills can be acquired and used by all members of the health care team but it is only when the client and a suitably trained counsellor agree to enter a counselling relationship that 'counselling' is said to be practised (BAC 1985).

## The counsellor and the treatment team

Clinicians, embryologists and nursing staff have roles to perform in treating the patient, helping the patient to understand the implications of each treatment and possible outcomes, administering the necessary drugs and carrying out surgical procedures. While involved in their roles they may also find themselves listening, empathising and responding helpfully to anxious, angry or grieving patients. The counsellor should be an integral part of the team approach and be easily accessible so that referral of patients, whether in a planned way or in a crisis scenario, can be achieved as simply as possible, perhaps by a brief letter, a personal communication, or a quick call on the extension. To be 'independent' does not necessarily mean to be based outside the unit. It may be taken to mean that the counsellor while playing his or her own professional role can understand but is not involved in the medical management of the patient. There is a need, therefore, for the counsellor to be fully aware of the process of treatment without necessarily becoming an expert on every aspect or meaning of the medical diagnosis. It also requires some self-learning on the part of the counsellor in relation to medical and scientific terminology and easy access to the clinicians to clarify any clinical information which may be important to understand before meeting with a client.

## Confidentiality and contract for counselling

Confidentiality is a delicate area. Both clinicians and counsellors have their own codes of conduct and confidentiality. To create a good and trusting working relationship it can be helpful if the counsellor draws up a document describing the agreement on confidentiality which will be held between the medical director, the counsellor and the patient. This can also include a clear 'contract for counselling', a clarification of the boundaries of responsibility, and the methods of referral which the counsellor would use especially in an emergency. After discussion and agreement this can be signed by both the medical director and the counsellor. A confidentiality agreement, in a simple form, between the patient and the counsellor can be signed by both patients and counsellor and then filed in the counselling file. A mutual feeling of trust can evolve through exploring these important aspects of the working relationship within the team, and this can lead to a respect for each other's professionalism.

Counselling should not be mandatory for treatment, but in some cases the counsellor may be asked to assess patients if there are aspects of their history or care which suggest to the clinician that they may benefit from counselling or

## Fertility counselling

the counsellor's opinion. It is important to make this clear to the patient before the session begins. There may also be ethical issues which indicate the patient's referral to the unit's ethics committee. The counsellor is not the best person to carry out the required in depth assessment as he or she may need to be involved with the care of the patient before and/or after the ethics committee decision. It would be more appropriate for another suitably qualified professional such as another counsellor or social worker or health psychologist to perform this duty.

### Counselling as part of treatment

Patients will be encouraged to ask for counselling if its availability is presented in a positive way by the clinician at an appropriate time, usually at their initial consultation. Many patients still confuse counselling with psychiatry and are very resistant to the idea. The service needs to be open and flexible, and receptive to referrals from anyone in the unit, and also from the patients themselves. Sometimes patients just need some extra time to understand the implications of what they are doing, or to use the counsellor as a 'bridge' to ask the questions they felt uncomfortable about asking the clinician directly.

### Counselling issues

People exhibit a broad spectrum of responses to the diagnosis of a fertility problem. While some seem to cope in a very practical way, others may be driven to despair and even contemplate suicide. The counsellor needs to have skills which will allow sensitive work to be carried out with couples, and women and men on their own. The counselling is usually short term and very intense. Occasionally a person, usually a woman, will return over a period of years in varying degrees of frequency according to whatever stage of treatment she has reached. The person's past family history, medical history, past and present relationships, previous losses and traumas can all be critical in terms of how an individual may cope with the present problem. Time is needed to unravel these important areas and listen to the individual's responses.

The stress of coping on a day to day basis with all the various hurdles of treatment is frequently overshadowed by an existential anxiety about the possibility of a childless future and a pervading sense of the meaninglessness of life and the unfairness of what is happening. There are very high levels of stress and anxiety, and a varying sense of depression as each individual tries to assimilate the relentless sensations of grief and loss after failed treatments. For example, pre-treatment obstetric and gynaecological losses, loss of embryos, the loss of opportunity especially felt by post-menopausal women and the loss of fertility felt by azoospermic men, all need to be addressed if the person is to be able to grieve and then accept the reality of the loss and begin to come to terms with the changed situation.

### Counselling for options

It appears that many couples would welcome counselling very early in their medical management, perhaps at the time when the anxiety was high enough for them to visit their family practitioner. Certainly an opportunity should be available as soon as a couple are referred to the general hospital infertility clinic and prior to any treatment beginning. Even so couples arrive at assisted conception units either without earlier counselling, or accepting counselling only when a crisis exists. During treatment a couple should be able to ask for counselling at any stage and team members need to be sensitive to those who may benefit but do not ask.

When treatment ends there can often be a void, an emptiness, a feeling of isolation and unsupportedness. Many people have indicated how they would have welcomed contact at this time. For those couples who realise that they have now no option but to end treatment this can be a time of grief once more. The counsellor can have a role here in supporting the couple and helping them to find their new role in life whether that be through adoption or remaining creatively childless. This is a time of parting, grieving, resolution and moving on. For some it can be a relief and they welcome the time to express this in the safety of the counselling relationship. Some marital relationships end at this stage and although the counsellor can be present for the couple it is good practice to refer the couple, if they so wish, to an appropriate local outside marital counselling agency.

### Counselling in relation to insemination with husband or donor semen

This is one part of the spectrum of treatment, but is often the starting point for many couples who are referred ultimately to assisted conception units. After listening to the clinician's explanation for the need for insemination many couples show reactions which parallel the recognised models of the tasks of mourning which are clearly described by Kubler-Ross (1973) and Worden (1991). The loss is all the more difficult to grieve over as it is an unseen loss, and much secrecy may exist about the treatment. In the counselling room there is the safety to feel the pain, open up the unspoken fears and move towards a time when decisions can be made which are acceptable to both partners so that their life can move on.

Fertility counselling is not long-term psychotherapy so essentially the counselling relationship needs to be more focused and short term and is constrained by the actual treatment time, or the accessibility of the patient to the counsellor. The Egan model of counselling (Egan 1986) is very helpful here as there are stages which can be easily defined such as (1) exploration of the situation and the feelings associated with the situation, (2) new understanding of the self, and (3) time for decision-making, acceptance and moving on. There is no opportunity to explore in depth this model of counselling and readers are referred to Egan (1986) and Mearns & Thorne (1988).

Many couples in treatment are apt to want everything to be medically focused. They come for diagnosis and treatment and when treatment fails they want to return as soon as possible to have more treatment. This cycle misses out the important aspect of attending to the couple's feelings and by not slowing down this process the welfare of the patients may be damaged. If treatment unfortunately fails, the ability to adjust to the long-term reality of childlessness may be extremely difficult for some people who have not had time to adjust to each loss and prepare themselves for the future (Read 1995).

### Issues related to male factor infertility and treatment by donor insemination

Studies have shown that almost 40% of fertility problems have a major male factor involvement, 40% will have a female factor and 20% will be a combination of both factors and unknown factors. In perhaps 50% of couples coming for treatment the male partner may be highly anxious about his own fertility. Few men come alone to see the counsellor, even though their female partners may come in a highly distressed state. The shock of being told he is infertile can be totally shattering and a man may experience a searing emotional reaction and grief. Men still find it difficult to talk about this to their family, friends and helping professionals. For those couples who are facing this problem the issues for counselling usually involve grief, a loss of identity as a man, a sense of uselessness and guilt, a need for clear information, confusion regarding the relationship between masculinity, fertility and sexuality, coming to terms with 'genetic death', the loss of self-esteem and self-image, the stress of treatment, a loss of intimacy, and perhaps sexual and relationship difficulties (Mason 1993; Entwhistle 1994). Within the counselling sessions there also needs to be time to explore the issues highlighted by the HFEA (1990) (Table 4.1).

Table 4.1. *Issues to be discussed in relation to donor insemination*

1. Concerns about using known/unknown donor sperm.
2. Who has been told of the problem?
3. How this will affect the couple's decision to tell the child.
4. The reasons (a) for telling the child, or (b) for not telling the child.
5. The need for privacy within the marriage.
6. How will they tell the child?
7. How will they handle it if the 'secret' is revealed inadvertently?
8. What scenarios may happen if the child finds out?
9. Fears of the male partner about his relationship with the child.
10. Facing the reality of the loss of a genetic future; what does this mean for each person?
11. Known donation: roles of the genetic/non-genetic parent
    boundaries which may need to exist or be created
    relationships in the future
12. Handling jealousy/envy.
13. If there is no conception/child, how do they feel?
14. If the child is born disabled or the foetus is abnormal; feelings then?
15. The role of the Central Register.
16. The health of the donor.
17. Anonymity of the donor.
18. Responsibilities of the donor and recipient parents.
19. The couple's awareness of the effects of bringing another child into the family if children from previous relationships already exist.
20. A need to clarify whether there are any reasons why relationships do not exist between the potential parents and previous children.
21. Exploring the possibility there may be a multiple pregnancy and the implications of this for the couple.
22. Allowing time for any further questions or issues.

### Counselling in relation to in vitro fertilisation and microassisted fertilisation

This often involves creating and maintaining a counselling relationship in depth and dealing with emotions, as previously described, but presented in a more extreme form as the couples will already have experienced the failure of previous treatments. Many seek in vitro fertilisation (IVF) as a last resort, knowing that the chances of success are restricted by opportunity, age and expense. At some point many couples will have to leave the unit knowing that nothing more can be done for them. This process can be very painful. Adoption may not be an option because the age limit has passed. The counsellor's role is to explore their understanding of the treatment, allowing expression of their grief, anger, denial, depression and anxiety, and helping the couple adjust to the reality of their situation. Many of the other previously discussed issues are also pertinent here. Women who have achieved the longed for pregnancy may find they are very anxious throughout the pregnancy, especially if there is need for prenatal testing of the foetus or there are added concerns of multiple pregnancy. They may wish to maintain contact with the counsellor during this period.

Increasingly couples are referred for IVF with donor sperm if there is a genetic problem in the family. Here, there are very special concerns which should have been addressed through the genetic counselling service but of which the counsellor needs to be aware. There may have been previous abortions, or stillbirths, or existing children who have inherited the condition. The counsellor may need to seek expert opinion or, with permission, to contact the referring hospital and speak to the genetic nurse specialist who has been in most contact with the couple. In this way a bridge is built which can support the couple as they leave one clinical situation and enter another with all the adjustments they may need to make within a new and stressful situation.

## Multicultural and religious issues

Most societies are, or are becoming, multiethnic. The team and the counsellor need to be aware of the cultural differences which may make treatment ethically difficult for patients. To discount others' belief systems and to be inflexible in administering treatment can only increase the stress for couples, especially women, who may also be coping with language and social isolation in a foreign country. An understanding of others' religious beliefs and an awareness of the couple's individual needs will ease the way for couples. Some couples may be seeking treatment which is diametrically opposed to their taught beliefs and this may become a dilemma of science versus religion to which it is difficult to become reconciled. If interpreters are used, there are additional issues of confidentiality to be considered between the couple, the interpreter and the counsellor. From time to time the counsellor may have to liaise with the hospital chaplains who tend to be receptive and sensitive to couples' difficulties, if this is acceptable to the couple. This added dimension of spirituality can be very calming to an emotionally distraught couple who are struggling to come to terms with a difficult personal decision. Other important members of the family may have to be involved in counselling sessions. In some ethnic groups, the mother-in-law can be a powerful influence in a household where several siblings have brought in wives, one of whom may have a fertility problem.

## Training, support and supervision of the counsellor

It is increasingly important that the counsellor has received adequate training for the complex role of fertility counsellor. This may mean having undertaken a recognised course of counsellor training which includes theory, practice and personal development in one or more of the main theoretical models of counselling. In addition there should be extra training in the specialism of fertility counselling. Local or national counselling associations and governmental regulatory bodies usually establish guidelines for good professional training to accepted standards. The counsellor needs to be adaptable and able to offer different techniques of counselling for different situations, for example crisis counselling and stress management. He or she also needs to be aware of the medical processes and current terminology.

In recognition of the stressful nature of fertility counselling, and because it is an essential part of the counselling ethos, the counsellor should receive clinical supervision on a regular basis from a qualified counselling supervisor, who is not a manager within the fertility unit. In addition the counsellor may seek personal support from other members of the unit with whom there is a working bond, or perhaps from the hospital chaplaincy. The counsellor may also choose to have his or her own personal therapy in order to challenge and understand the emotional reactions arising from fertility work and to bring about a deeper self-understanding.

## Conclusion

Fertility counselling is a new specialism within the counselling profession. At present many fertility units and the people within them are working towards creating a mutually respectful environment for the psychological, emotional and spiritual welfare of their patients. The counsellor's role is that of an emotional support service for patients who find their treatment highly stressful. This role may encompass offering support to the staff working in the unit. In addition the counsellor should have access to an internal and external network of referral agencies to whom the patients can be helpfully guided when necessary. Lastly, the counsellor should be appropriately trained, with on-going clinical supervision and be accepted as one of the team in the care and treatment of patients. There will be many different ways of achieving this and the present account has described one of them.

**References**

British Association for Counselling. (1985) *Code of Ethics and Practice for Counsellors*.

Egan R. (1986) *The Skilled Helper,* third edition. Brookes/Cole Publishing Company, Monterus, California.
Entwhistle P. (1994) Counselling in male fertility. *Journal of Fertilty Counselling* **1,** 7–10.
Human Fertilisation and Embryology Authority. (1990) *Code of Practice.* London, pp. 28–29.
Kubler-Ross E. (1973) *On Death and Dying.* Tavistock Press, London.
Mason M. C. (1993) *Male Infertility – Men Talking.* Routledge, London.
Mearns D. & Thorne B. (1988) *Person-Centred Counselling In Action.* Sage Publications Ltd, London.
Read J. (1995) *Counselling for Fertility Problems.* Sage Publications Ltd, London.
Sanders P. (1994) *First Steps in Counselling.* PCCS Books, Manchester, p. 10.
Worden W. J. (1991) *Grief Counselling and Grief Therapy: A Handbook for the Practitioner,* second edition. Routledge, London.

**Recommended reading**

Egan R. (1986) *The Skilled Helper,* third edition. Brookes/Cole Publishing Company, Monterus, California.
Jennings S. E. (ed.) (1995) *Infertility Counselling.* Blackwell Science Ltd, Oxford.
Mason M. C.(1993) *Male Infertility – Men Talking.* Routledge, London.
Mearns D. & Thorne B. (1988) *Person-Centred Counselling In Action.* Sage Publications Ltd, London.
Read J. (1995) *Counselling for Fertility Problems.* Sage Publications Ltd, London.
Rogers C. R. (1951) *Client-Centred Therapy.* Constable and Co. Ltd, London.
Rogers C. R. (1961) *On Becoming A Person.* Constable and Co. Ltd, London.
Snowden R. & Snowden E. (1993) *The Gift Of A Child. A Guide To Donor Insemination.* University of Exeter Press, Exeter.

# 5

# Ovarian stimulation for the assisted reproduction technologies

GODWIN I. MENIRU and IAN L. CRAFT

**Introduction**

The birth of Louise Brown on 28 July 1978 (Steptoe & Edwards 1978) marked the beginning of an era of rapid expansion in the scope of treatment options available to infertile couples, as well as an improvement of their success rate. With these advances came the establishment of assisted reproduction technology as the ultimate scientific and clinical tool, enabling a large proportion of infertile couples to achieve the supreme aspiration of many couples existing in stable relationships. A key requirement for most assisted conception treatments is the stimulation of multiple follicular development and the production of many mature oocytes, as this is generally associated with improved chances of conception. This is unlike induction of ovulation where the aim is usually to mimic the normal growth and eventual release of an oocyte from the dominant follicle. Different terminology have been used by various workers when describing the type of ovarian stimulation carried out during assisted conception treatment and include superovulation, superovulation induction, controlled hyperstimulation of the ovary, ovarian hyperstimulation, induction of ovulation and controlled ovarian superovulation (Devroey et al. 1992a). A number of pharmacological preparations and stimulation protocols have been tried with each having its peculiar methodology, dosage regimens, merits and shortcomings. These and related issues will be examined in the following sections which start with a description of drugs of interest (Tables 5.1 and 5.2), followed by discussions relating to methods of superovulation. It is hoped that this chapter will form a suitable introduction to the next one, where ovarian stimulation for intrauterine insemination will be considered specifically.

Table 5.1. *Superovulation agents*

| Agent | Trade name | Company |
| --- | --- | --- |
| *Anti-oestrogens* | | |
| Clomiphene citrate | Clomid | Merrell |
| | Serophene | Serono |
| Cyclofenil | Rehibin | Serono |
| Tamoxifen | Nolvadex | ICI |
| *Gonadotrophins* | | |
| hMG | Humegon (FSH:LH = 1:1) | Organon |
| | Normegon (FSH:LH = 3:1) | Organon |
| | Pergonal (FSH:LH = 1:1) | Serono |
| 'Pure' FSH | Metrodin, Metrodin 'High' Purity | Serono |
| | Orgafol | Organon |
| hCG | Gonadotraphon | Paines and Byrne |
| | Pregnyl | Organon |
| | Profasi | Serono |
| Recombinant FSH | Gonal-F | Serono |
| | Puregon | Organon |

Table 5.2. *Gonadotrophin releasing hormone agonists currently used in superovulation regimens*

| Agonist | Trade name | Company | Route |
| --- | --- | --- | --- |
| Buserelin | Suprecur | Hoechst | N |
| | Suprefact | Hoechst | N/SC |
| Goserelin | Zoladex | ICI | SC-implant |
| Leuprorelin | Prostap SR | Lederle–Takeda | SC/IM |
| Naferelin | Synarel | Syntex | N |
| Triptorelin | Decapeptyl | Salk/Ferring | SC-implant |

*Notes:*
SC: subcutaneous; IM: intramuscular; N: intranasal.

## Agents utilised during superovulation

### *Clomiphene citrate*

This non-steroidal triphenylethylene derivative, which has some structural similarities with diethylstilboestrol (Figure 5.1), came into clinical use in the 1960s (Chen & Wallach 1994). It is probably the most extensively utilised drug

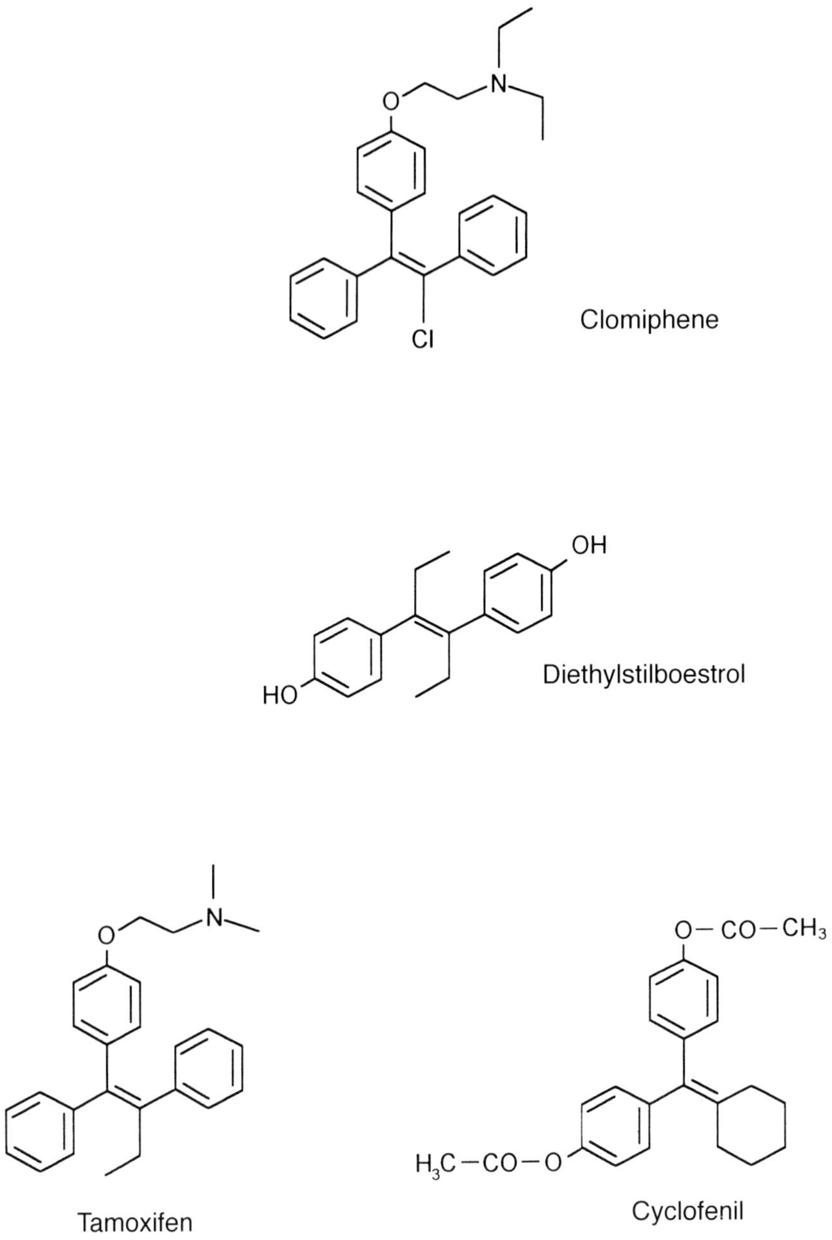

Figure 5.1. Clomiphene and related compounds.

for ovulation induction with more than 4951 reports pertaining to its use having been published in scientific journals at the last count (Lunenfeld & Insler 1990). Clomiphene citrate has mainly anti-oestrogenic properties but it also exhibits mild oestrogenic activity in certain situations (Taubet & Kuhl

*Ovarian stimulation for assisted reproduction* 59

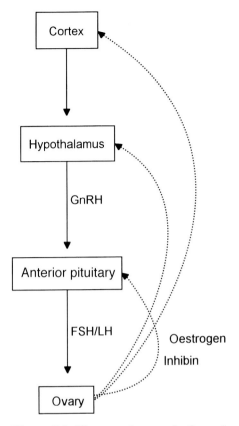

Figure 5.2. Hormonal control of ovarian function. FSH: follicle stimulating hormone; GnRH: gonadotrophin releasing hormone; LH: luteinising hormone.

1994). Clomiphene citrate competes with oestrogen for pituitary and probably hypothalamic and ovarian binding sites (van Uem & Hodgen 1986; Taubet & Kuhl 1994). Successful interaction with these receptors interrupts the negative feedback action of endogenous oestrogen levels (Figure 5.2) and this results in an increased output of gonadotrophin releasing hormone (GnRH) from the hypothalamus. GnRH in turn stimulates release of follicle stimulating hormone (FSH) and luteinising hormone (LH) from the anterior pituitary gland. Increased levels of FSH and LH lead to recruitment of more follicles which together produce greater amounts of oestrogen (Lunenfeld & Insler 1990). The net effect of this enhancement of ovarian activity is that of an increased chance of ovulation of more than one mature follicle. Similar drugs such as cyclofenil and tamoxifen have not enjoyed as much popularity as clomiphene citrate. Cyclofenil is administered at a dose of 200 mg three times daily for 5 days while tamoxifen is administered at the dose of 20 mg once daily also for 5 days. Just like clomiphene citrate, administration of these drugs is commenced in the early follicular phase of the menstrual cycle following onset of a menstrual period or withdrawal bleeding.

### *Gonadotrophins*

Administration of exogenous gonadotrophins increases the number of follicles recruited into the growing pool and maintains their growth until the stage of ovulation. Cole and Hart first reported in 1930, their attempts to induce ovulation in laboratory animals using extracts from pregnant mare serum (Chen & Wallach 1994). Gonadotrophins from pituitary and urinary extracts of humans and animals were also used in subsequent years but the rapid development of antibodies to preparations from non-primate animal sources militated against their continued usage because the desired clinical effects were neutralised by these antibodies. Many women who received human pituitary extracts of these hormones have since died from Creutzfeld–Jakob disease.

Human menopausal gonadotrophin (hMG) came into use in the 1960s. It is produced by extracting gonadotrophins from the urine of menopausal women and contains equal proportions of FSH and LH. Other preparations containing FSH with reduced or virtually no LH, were later introduced as a result of the hypothesis that tonically elevated plasma LH concentrations found especially in women with polycystic ovarian syndrome were mainly responsible for the suboptimal outcome of ovulation induction in these females; these women probably needed only exogenous FSH as endogenous LH levels would be sufficient for the completion of follicular development.

Recombinant FSH is prepared from cultures of Chinese hamster ovarian cells and is now available for routine clinical use. Part of the impetus behind this development has been the fact that other gonadotrophin preparations are contaminated with variable amounts of urinary proteins and other compounds, and exhibit wide batch to batch variability in the content and biological activity of gonadotrophins. Moreover, the rapid increase in demand for gonadotrophin preparations put a severe strain on the supply of postmenopausal urine. The manufacturing process of recombinant FSH is more efficient and there is virtually no fear of disease transmission to patients. Recombinant gonadotrophins are of high purity, have specific activity, are safe and effective (Mannaerts *et al.* 1991, 1993; Devroey *et al.* 1994). Since the early reports of pregnancies and deliveries following the use of this preparation were made (Devroey *et al.* 1992a,b; Donderwinkel *et al.* 1992; Germond *et al.* 1992) several more babies have been born.

Recombinant LH will hopefully also become available for clinical use.

Meanwhile, human chorionic gonadotrophin (hCG), which has predominantly luteinising properties (Walker 1993), is still being extracted from the urine of pregnant women. It is injected in doses of between 5000 and 10,000 IU when the growing follicles reach the required diameter. This leads to maturation of the oocytes within the follicles and commencement of ovulation about 37 hours later.

### Gonadotrophin releasing hormone and its agonists

Schally and Guillemin independently isolated and characterised the structure of luteinising hormone-releasing hormone (LHRH) with their workers in 1971 (Howles 1990; Lunenfeld & Insler 1990; Chen & Wallach 1994). GnRH is used synonymously with LHRH and is a short acting 10-amino acid polypeptide which is secreted by the hypothalamus at the rate of one pulse per hour (Elkind-Hirsch et al. 1982). Agonists of GnRH (GnRHa) were synthesised later on in order to increase the half-life of the drug. This was achieved by substituting amino acid molecules in the native compound with other amino acids or more complex molecules (Figure 5.3).

Commercially available preparations commonly have the substitution at position 6, and at times position 10, of the natural peptide (Howles 1990). These agonists have a greater affinity for the GnRH receptor, are less subject to enzyme degradation, have a longer half-life of 80 minutes and have up to 50–100 times the potency of GnRH. Results of ovulation induction were initially disappointing as the significance of the pulsatile manner of GnRH secretion was not appreciated. It was only after Knobil's (1980) work with pulsatile administration of GnRH to monkeys with lesioned hypothalami, that real progress began to be made in the use of this compound and its analogues for the induction of ovulation in women with ovulatory dysfunction.

The manner of action which is utilised in assisted conception treatments differs from the above. When an agonist is given initially it causes release of LH and FSH from the pituitary in amounts similar to those found during the midcycle LH surge. Chronic frequent administration leads to a decrease and finally virtual abolition of further secretion as the pituitary becomes insensitive to additional stimulation. This phenomenon which is usually noted by the fourth day of administration (Fleming et al. 1990; Howles 1990) is caused by the loss of occupied GnRH receptors on the surface of pituitary gonadotrope cells (called downregulation) and uncoupling of the receptors from the secretory signal (called desensitisation) (Howles 1990).

Secretion of LH and FSH by the pituitary does not cease completely but continues at baseline levels except for possibly in the case of depot agonist

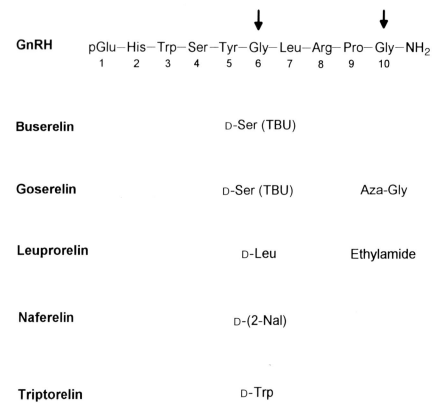

Figure 5.3. Gonadotrophin releasing hormone (GnRH) and substituted groups in agonists commonly used in superovulation regimens.

administration where a more profound suppression of gonadotrophin secretion occurs. The important effect of agonist use is that the LH surge is prevented from occurring. Endogenous gonadotrophin secretory patterns, however, return rapidly to normal as soon as the GnRHa is discontinued. The use of buserelin in conjunction with hMG was first reported in 1984 by Porter and colleagues. Most units have now incorporated these drugs into their superovulation protocols. Some use GnRHa only in special groups of patients such as poor responders (Cummins *et al.* 1989) while others use them for all patients (Tan 1994).

## Superovulation methods

### Monitoring

Monitoring of patient response can be carried out with a combination of ultrasound scanning of the ovaries and uterine endometrium, and assay of the serum concentration of LH, FSH, progesterone and oestrogen. These tests are carried out at different intervals both before and during superovulation. Not all parameters are checked at every monitoring episode, and various units have their own particular protocols for such tests. Broadly speaking, patients are usually checked before commencing superovulation to exclude any pathology that contraindicates the proposed treatment or requires its modification. Assessment at this period also aims to confirm that the patient's physiology is what it should be at that part of the ovarian cycle.

Response to treatment is assessed during the period of ovarian stimulation to confirm its adequacy. Suboptimal responses call for alteration of the drug treatment protocol or cancellation of the treatment cycle. Such checks will also help decide on when to schedule hCG administration and oocyte retrieval or artificial insemination. Complications of the treatment procedure are also sought for especially at their early stages so that measures can be taken to prevent their occurrence or further deterioration, and to treat established cases. It is becoming increasingly clear that assisted conception treatments can be safely monitored with ultrasound scanning alone (Smith *et al.* 1984; Golan *et al.* 1994; Tsirigotis *et al.* 1995). This policy is still compatible with normal pregnancy rates and a low incidence of the ovarian hyperstimulation syndrome.

### *Sole use of clomiphene citrate*

Following the first few natural cycle in vitro fertilisation (IVF) pregnancies it became obvious that this was an inefficient way of conducting assisted conception programmes because of the requirement for intense patient monitoring. Furthermore, outcome of treatment depended solely on the integrity of a single gamete. Lopata is credited with the first attempts at inducing multiple follicular development with clomiphene citrate for IVF during the 1970s (Ron-El *et al.* 1993) but it was Trounson and his co-workers (1981) who demonstrated that multiple follicular development could be reliably induced with clomiphene citrate and the oocytes programmed for aspiration 35–36 hours following an injection of hCG. The dose of clomiphene citrate was between 100 and 150 mg and this was administered daily for 5 days. Pregnancy rates were not improved by giving lower doses or increasing the number of days of administration (Marrs *et al.* 1983). Commencement of clomiphene citrate on day 5 of the cycle gave the best results. Starting treatment on day 3 increased the incidence of poor response from 3% to 35% (Ron-El *et al.* 1993). Starting it on day 7 led to an increase in the incidence of a single dominant follicle to 23%, which is not surprising when it is remembered that selection of the dominant follicle and atresia of the rest of the recruited follicles occur relatively early in the menstrual cycle. The incidence of spontaneous LH surges varied with the day of starting therapy with clomiphene citrate such that it was 8, 2 and 10% for commencement of clomiphene citrate on days 3, 5 and 7, respectively (Marrs *et al.* 1984).

The long running controversy regarding the possible deleterious effects of clomiphene citrate on reproductive function also surfaced here. While clomiphene citrate was blamed for having detrimental effects on the quality of follicular fluid, oocytes, endometrium and luteal phase, no report came out with categorical proof of an association (Ron-El *et al.* 1993). The lower pregnancy rate associated with the use of clomiphene citrate alone, when compared with that obtained with gonadotrophins, is most probably due to the smaller number of follicles that hormonal changes induced by clomiphene citrate can recruit and maintain. This means that there will be a reduced number of embryos available for transfer. The sole use of clomiphene citrate for superovulation has been abandoned in most IVF units.

## *Combined use of clomiphene citrate and gonadotrophins*

A combination regimen of clomiphene citrate and hMG came into use as a method of ovarian stimulation in the early 1980s. This entails the administration of 50–100 mg of clomiphene citrate for 5 days starting from days 2, 3, 4 or 5 depending on the previous menstrual cycle lengths and experience of the clinician in charge. hMG is started on the last day of administering clomiphene citrate, or a few days before that, at a dose of 150–225 IU per day, depending on the size of the growing follicles. It is continued until at least one follicle reaches 18 mm in diameter. hCG is given 36–48 hours after the last dose of hMG. This method was associated with an improvement of the pregnancy rate per transfer to 38% compared to the previous rate of 15% for single agent treatment (Lopata 1983). More oocytes were retrieved and this led to an increased number of embryos being available for transfer. There were still problems with this method of stimulation. A cycle cancellation rate of 25% was quoted by Taymor *et al.* (1985) and this was due to premature LH surges, poor oestradiol profiles, poor response and inadequate follicular development.

Despite these problems, pregnancy rates of 18–20% associated with the use of clomiphene citrate/hMG compared favourably with those of other regimens reported in the 1989 and 1990 IVF register for the USA (Medical Research International 1991, 1992). Use of the clomiphene citrate/FSH protocol has not been popular although it has similar cancellation, fertilisation and conception rates with the clomiphene citrate/hMG combination (Quigley *et al.* 1988). All regimens that included clomiphene citrate have largely been superseded by those using gonadotrophins alone or with GnRHa, however, because of cost considerations, some centres in poorer economies may continue to use clomiphene citrate either alone or in combination with gonadotrophins.

### Sole use of gonadotrophins

Jones *et al.* (1982) were one of the first groups to use gonadotrophins for superovulation. Daily administration of hMG was commenced on day 3 of the menstrual cycle and serial assays of serum oestradiol concentration started from day 6 together with ovarian ultrasound scans. hMG was stopped when a follicle measured 12 mm or more and 10 000 IU of hCG administered 50–52 hours later. Oocyte retrieval took place 35–36 hours from the time of the hCG injection.

The interval between the last dose of hMG and the injection of hCG was shortened to 28–30 hours in certain situations: (1) the leading follicle measured 16 mm or above in diameter, (2) plateau or doubling of the oestradiol level when compared to the previous day's level, and (3) beginning of an LH surge. This group of workers later published their findings on the association of oestrogen profiles during follicular stimulation and outcome of the treatment cycle (Jones *et al.* 1983). Recognition of these patterns assisted individualisation of treatment schedules. The same group (Bernardus *et al.* 1985) described the beneficial effects of supplementing hMG administration with that of FSH on the first 2 days of the stimulation cycle in women with poor ovarian responses in previous cycles.

Sole use of FSH was reported by Jones *et al.* (1985) but prospective randomised studies (Scoccia *et al.* 1987) and the data from the IVF registry in America (Medical Research International 1991, 1992) showed no differences in the pregnancy rate between the hMG and hMG/FSH protocols (Ron-El *et al.* 1993). Scoccia *et al.* (1987), however, found lower cancellation rates when FSH was used alone. Spontaneous LH surges have remained a troublesome factor in superovulation regimens already described and are probably the major reason why many units now use some or all of the protocols to be described in the following section.

### Routine use of gonadotrophin releasing hormone agonists during superovulation with gonadotrophins

Inclusion of GnRHa in regimens for superovulation has largely removed the problem of spontaneous LH surge and it now occurs in less than 3% of cycles (Caspi *et al.* 1989; MacLachlan *et al.* 1989). A net increase in the pregnancy

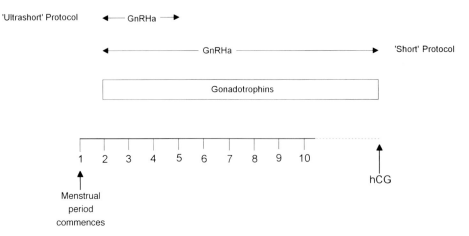

Figure 5.4. 'Short' and 'ultrashort' protocols of ovarian stimulation. GnRHa: gonadotrophin releasing hormone agonist; hCG: human chorionic gonadotrophin.

rate per cycle has also occurred (Neveu et al. 1987). Women who previously showed a poor response with other regimens now have better results (Cummins et al. 1989). Pregnancy rates in women with moderate to severe endometriosis seem to be higher too (Oehninger et al. 1989; Dicker et al. 1990). There is still controversy as to whether the suppression of tonically elevated plasma LH concentration found in women with polycystic ovarian syndrome improves outcome of assisted conception treatment in such females (Salat-Baroux et al. 1988; Owen et al. 1989). Patients with incipient ovarian failure will not be helped by inclusion of GnRHa and probably need to be identified beforehand (Ron-El et al. 1993) and offered alternative management options.

GnRHa is currently used in three ways during superovulation and these have been given the names 'long', 'short' and 'ultrashort' protocols (Figures 5.4 and 5.5). In the long protocol, administration of the agonist is commenced on day 21 of the previous menstrual cycle or day 1 or 2 of the present cycle (i.e. treatment cycle) and continued till the day of hCG administration (Tan 1994). If commenced on day 1 of the woman's cycle, at least 10–14 days should be allowed to elapse for adequate pituitary desensitisation to occur before commencing gonadotrophin injections. The dose of GnRHa can be reduced by half once pituitary desensitisation is confirmed (Meldrum et al. 1988). This is understandably not possible in cases where depot GnRHa injection is administered. The short protocol involves starting the administration of GnRHa anytime within the first 3 days of the menstrual (treatment) cycle and adding gonadotrophin injections after 1 or 2 days. The agonist is continued until the day of hCG administration. The ultrashort protocol differs from the short type

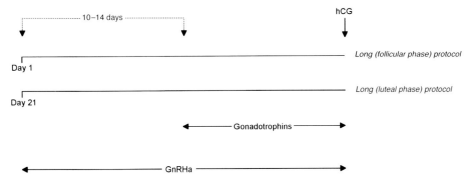

Figure 5.5. Ovarian stimulation using variants of the long protocol. GnRHa: gonadotrophin releasing hormone agonist; hCG: human chorionic gonadotrophin.

mainly because administration of GnRHa is limited to 3 days (Howles *et al.* 1987).

The relative merits of these treatment regimens have been the source of much controversy. While the long protocol aims at suppression of ovarian activity before commencing gonadotrophin injections, the initial discharge of endogenous gonadotrophins by the pituitary at the beginning of agonist administration, called the 'flare-up' phenomenon, is utilised in the other two protocols in order to facilitate follicular recruitment (Howles 1990) and decrease the total amount of exogenous gonadotrophin administered in the treatment cycle thereby reducing costs. Short protocols have been criticised on a number of grounds. The 'flare-up' phenomenon may lead to rescue of the corpus luteum of the previous cycle which then causes inappropriate progesterone secretion (Howles *et al.* 1987) and thecal androgen production (Stanger & Yovich 1985; Howles *et al.* 1986) in the follicular phase of the treatment cycle. Luteinisation of developing antral follicles is also possible due to the high levels of LH during the 'flare-up' period. Ovarian ultrasound scanning and progesterone assay at the beginning of agonist administration may reveal cases with persisting corpora lutea or elevated progesterone levels. GnRHa administration can then be continued in these women until the ovary becomes quiescent before commencing gonadotrophin administration (Howles 1990). An alternative would be to bring about quiescence of the ovary by giving norethisterone tablets (Primolut N; Schering Health Care, West Sussex, UK) from day 2 of the previous cycle and continue for 7–25 days before starting the short protocols (Zorn *et al.* 1987). Another problem with the use of short protocols is that endogenous gonadotrophin levels may not fall to the expected low levels during the period of follicular stimulation (Howles 1990). This becomes more important in women with tonically high LH levels who actually take a longer time to reach adequate pituitary desensitisation (Fleming *et al.* 1982). Premature LH surges can also occur in 5–10% of short protocol cycles.

Major attributes of the long protocol include the decreased need for intensive monitoring and the fact that it allows flexibility in scheduling the commencement of gonadotrophin injections and the time for oocyte recovery. Increase in costs due to the utilisation of greater amounts of agonists, because of the longer duration of use and possibly a greater requirement for exogenous gonadotrophins, appear initially to be strong points against this type of protocol. When savings made from decreased cancellation rates and higher pregnancy rates (Tan 1994) are taken into consideration, however, this line of argument becomes less persuasive. It has to be reiterated that this protocol is more convenient and associated with less administrative problems and out of hours work activity in the unit concerned. A further advantage in the use of the long protocol is that in situations of asynchronous follicular growth during superovulation, the fact that spontaneous surge of LH has been prevented, allows for prolongation of the stimulatory period in order for more follicles to reach the desired size before hCG is administered (Tan 1994).

A recent meta-analysis of randomised and quasi-randomised studies by Hughes *et al.* (1992) confirmed that GnRHa reduced cycle cancellation rates, increased both the number of oocytes retrieved and the clinical pregnancy rates per cycle commenced and per embryo transfer. Tan (1994) referred to another study which was in press. This involved 2900 women who had one out of five regimens and remained with the chosen method throughout their treatment cycles. The five regimens were: (1) hMG – clomiphene citrate, (2) FSH – clomiphene citrate, (3) ultrashort protocol, (4) short protocol, and (5) long protocol. The agonist used was buserelin. He and his co-workers found that women who had the long protocol had significantly higher cumulative conception and livebirth rates when compared to women in the other groups. It should however be realised that specific patients may respond optimally and become pregnant with one of the short protocols having previously had poor results with the long protocol.

Fear has been expressed in various quarters regarding possible deleterious effects of these agonists on embryo quality and teratogenicity especially as it is realised that depot injections, for example, may still not be exhausted by the time of embryo implantation and early pregnancy. No teratogenic effects have been noted so far in humans and other mammalian species (Howles 1990). Thawed embryos which had been frozen at the pronuclear stage showed similar developmental patterns when related to use or non-use of GnRHa during superovulation with gonadotrophins (Oehninger 1992). The long protocol using buserelin has actually been found to be associated with a lower miscarriage rate of 20.3% as compared to the rate of 47.2% found when clomiphene citrate was used in women with polycystic ovarian syndrome (Balen *et al.* 1992).

### *Adjunctive use of growth hormone during superovulation*

Recent evidence suggests that administration of growth hormone (GH) preparations during superovulation, especially in certain groups of patients, may improve the outcome of different aspects of assisted conception treatment (Katz 1993). If this association is real, the effect could be mediated through the interaction of GH with ovarian GH receptors and/or by stimulation of insulin-like growth factor gene expression in the ovary. In doing so GH amplifies both endogenous and exogenous gonadotrophin activity on the ovary. The effect of different doses of GH and intervals of administration have been examined in various classes of women undergoing superovulation. The predominant finding is that of significant reduction of the duration of treatment and the daily effective dose of gonadotrophin, increased number of oocytes collected and improvement of fertilisation rates (Blumfeld & Lunenfeld 1989; Homburg *et al.* 1990; Volpe *et al.* 1990). This enhancement of response persisted in subsequent cycles in which superovulation was carried out without adjunctive use of GH (Burger *et al.* 1991). These beneficial effects have not been found in all studies or women tested (Katz 1993). The task for the future is for continued evaluation of this important finding so as to determine the exact mechanism of GH action on the ovary. This will hopefully help to delineate groups of patients who will benefit from GH administration during superovulation and refine our understanding of dosage requirements.

### *Complications of superovulation methods*

The superovulation methods are intensive and expose the patient to substantial emotional stress. These women have to endure numerous needle pricks from injections and withdrawal of blood specimens for various tests and repeated hormone assays. There is some degree of disruption of their social and work schedule as they have to report to hospital several times during the treatment period. Some may find transvaginal ultrasound scans aesthetically unappealing but put up with it as they realise the importance of such techniques. Despite all personal sacrifices a large majority of couples will have disappointed expectations in each cycle of treatment; current successes have not exceeded 30% per cycle on the average. The most common medical complication is that of ovarian cysts which usually appear at the initial phase of treatment with GnRHa (Remohi & Pellicer 1993). The incidence is between 14 and 29% (Feldberg et al. 1989; Ron-El et al. 1989; Sampaio et al. 1991) and are more frequent with short protocols (23%) than with long protocols (10%) (Sampaio et al. 1991). This suggests that these cysts are given rise to by the 'flare-up' phenomenon. They do not increase further in size during the rest of the treatment cycle and do not seem to affect the outcome of IVF (Ron-El et al. 1989).

Ovarian hyperstimulation syndrome is the most serious immediate complication of ovarian stimulation and the incidence is highest in cycles employing GnRHa (Tan 1994). Women with polycystic ovarian syndrome are at a higher risk of having this problem. While there is some element of hyperstimulation in most women having superovulation, the incidence of the severe variety has been put at 8.4% (Golan et al. 1988). The reason for the greater association with GnRHa administration is not known but it is most likely to derive from the fact that premature LH surges, which previously meant cancellation of cycles using earlier treatment protocols, are now abolished with the use of agonists and so one of the body's protective mechanisms against excessive ovarian activity is removed. The management of many of these complications will be discussed in a later chapter.

Multiple pregnancy is not a direct complication of superovulation but the ability to induce multiple follicular development means that there is an increased chance of more than one embryo implanting in the uterine cavity. Several complications are possible in multiple pregnancies, chief among which is premature labour and delivery.

Some worry has been expressed regarding a possible association between ovulation induction and the later development of ovarian malignancies (Fishel & Jackson 1989; Goldberg & Runowicz 1992; Willemsen et al. 1993). This is a highly charged topic in fertility management (Whittemore et al. 1992; Balasch & Barri 1993; Cohen et al. 1993; Sassoon 1993; Whittemore 1993) but issues will not be helped by publication of results of poorly designed studies or hasty attempts by others to discredit available, albeit tenuous, evidence. If there is a cause–effect relationship, it could be of two types; an early effect which takes the form of rapid growth of pre-existing tumours caused by increased ovarian vascular perfusion and altered hormonal milieu brought about by the administered gonadotrophins. The late effect may be due to carcinogenic substances arising from the large doses of gonadotrophins or their breakdown products, or the effect of multiple follicular development and ovulation stimulated by these drugs. Most interventions employed in assisted conception treatments are relatively new in medical science and it is only with time that present apparently safe techniques can be confirmed to be so. Meanwhile, continuous audit of results and monitoring of the future welfare of all participants and offspring of this program will go a long way towards resolving the dispute.

**Conclusion**

The advent of powerful agents for superovulation and the ability to prevent spontaneous surges of LH are some of the major reasons for recent increases in the success of assisted conception treatments. There is still room for improvement in a number of areas. Agents and methods for finer control of ovarian stimulation are needed to decrease the problem of ovarian hyperstimulation syndrome and the possible deleterious effects of medications on both gamete quality and the subsequent welfare of these women. The availability of recombinant FSH and LH would allow a more precise control of dosage requirements (Kempers 1994). More convenient routes and intervals of administration should be explored so as to reduce the stress, and possibly, costs of these procedures.

The development of potent GnRH antagonists has been slow and problematic due to a number of factors which were discussed by Howles (1990). These compounds will be useful for at least certain classes of patients especially those in whom the initial upsurge of endogenous gonadotrophin is to be avoided. Their introduction will also mean a fundamental change in present stimulation protocols. Finally, developments in other areas, especially in terms of maximising optimal conditions for embryo implantation and survival and treatment of male infertility, may make it unnecessary for the induction of multiple follicular development. The ability to culture immature oocytes successfully in vitro and even cryopreserve them could have the same effect on the requirement for superovulation.

**References**

Balasch J. & Barri P. N. (1993) Follicular stimulation and ovarian cancer? *Human Reproduction* **8**, 990–996.

Balen A., Tan S. L., MacDougall M. J. & Jacobs H. S. (1992) Miscarriage rates following in-vitro fertilisation are increased in women with polycystic ovaries and reduced by pituitary desensitisation with buserelin. *Human Reproduction* **8**, 959–964.

Bernardus R. E., Jones G. S., Acosta A. A., Garcia J. E., Liu H. C., Jones D. L. & Rosenwaks Z. (1985) The significance of the ratio in follicle stimulating hormone and luteinising hormone in induction of multiple follicular growth. *Fertility and Sterility* **43**, 373–378.

Blumfeld Z. & Lunenfeld B. (1989) The potentiating effect of growth hormone on follicle stimulation with human menopausal gonadotrophins in a panhypopituitary patient. *Fertility and Sterility* **52**, 328–331.

Burger H. G., Kovacs G. T., Polson D. M., McDonald J., McCloud P. I., Harrop M., Colman P. & Healy D. L. (1991) Ovarian sensitization to gonadotrophins by human growth hormone: persistence of effect beyond the treated cycle. *Clinical Endocrinology* **35**, 119–122.

Caspi E., Ron-El R., Golan A., Nachum H., Herman A., Soffer Y. & Weinraub Z. (1989) Results of *in vitro* fertilization and embryo transfer by combined long-acting gonadotropin-releasing hormone analog D-Trp-6 luteinizing hormone-releasing hormone and gonadotropins. *Fertility and Sterility* **51**, 95–99.

Chen S. H. & Wallach E. E. (1994) Five decades of progress in management of the infertile couple. *Fertility and Sterility* **62**, 665–685.

Cohen J., Forman R., Harlap S., Johannison E., Lunenfeld B., de Mouzon J., Pepperell R., Tarlatzis B. & Templeton A. (1993) IFFS expert group report on the Whittemore study related to the risk of ovarian cancer associated with the use of infertility agents. *Human Reproduction* **8**, 996–999.

Cummins J. M., Yovich J. M., Edinsinghe W. R. & Yovich J. L. (1989) Pituitary down-regulation using leuprolide for the intensive ovulation management of poor prognosis patients having in vitro fertilization (ivf) related treatments. *Journal of In Vitro Fertilization and Embryo Transfer* **6**, 345–352.

Devroey P., Mannaerts B., Smitz J., Coelingh Bennink H. & Van Steirteghem A. (1994) Clinical outcome of a pilot efficacy study on recombinant human follicle-stimulating hormone (Org 32489) combined with various gonadotrophin-releasing hormone agonist regimens. *Human Reproduction* **9**, 1064–1069.

Devroey P., Van Steirteghem A., Mannaerts B. & Bennink H. C. (1992a) Successful in vitro fertilisation and embryo transfer after treatment with recombinant human FSH. *Lancet* **339**, 1170–1171.

Devroey P., Van Steirteghem A., Mannaerts B. & Bennink H. C. (1992b) First singleton term birth after ovarian superovulation with rhFSH. *Lancet* **340**, 1108–1109.

Donderwinkel P. F. J., Schoot D. C., Coelingh Bennink H. J. T. & Fauser B. C. J. M. (1992) Pregnancy after induction of ovulation with recombinant human FSH in polycystic ovary syndrome. *Lancet* **340**, 983.

Dicker D., Goldman G. A., Ashkenazi J., Feldberg D., Voliovitz I. & Goldman J. A. (1990) The value of pretreatment with gonadotrophin releasing hormone (GnRH) analogue in IVF-ET therapy of severe endometriosis. *Human Reproduction* **5**, 418.

Elkind-Hirsch K., Schiff I., Ravnikar V., Tulchinsky D. & Ryan K. J. (1982) Determinations of endogenous immunoreactive luteinizing hormone releasing hormone in human plasma. *Journal of Clinical Endocrinology and Metabolism* **54**, 602–607.

Feldberg D., Ashkenazi J., Dicker D., Yeshaya A., Goldman G. A., Dicker D. & Goldman J. A. (1989) Ovarian cyst formation: a complication of gonadotropin hormone-releasing hormone agonist therapy. *Fertility and Sterility* **51**, 42–45.

Fishel S. & Jackson P. (1989) Follicular stimulation for high tech pregnancies: are we playing it safe? *British Medical Journal* **299**, 309–311.

Fleming R., Adam A. H., Barlow D. H., Black W. P., MacNaughton M. C. & Coutts J. R. (1982) A new systematic treatment for infertile women with abnormal hormone profiles. *British Journal of Obstetrics and Gynaecology* **89**, 80–83.

Fleming R., Jamieson M. E. & Coutts J. R. T. (1990) The use of GnRH-analogs in assisted reproduction. In: *Clinical IVF Forum*. (P. L. Matson, B. A. Lieberman, eds), Manchester University Press, Manchester, pp. 1–19.

Germond M., Dessole S., Senn A., Loumaye E., Howles C. & Beltrami V. (1992) Successful in vitro fertilisation and embryo transfer after treatment with recombinant human FSH. *Lancet* **339**, 1170 (letter).

Golan A., Herman A., Soffer Y., Bukovsky I. & Ron-El R. (1994) Ultrasonic control without hormone determination for ovulation induction in in-vitro fertilization/embryo transfer with gonadotrophin-releasing hormone analogue and human menopausal gonadotrophin. *Human Reproduction* **9**, 1631–1633.

Golan A., Ron-El R., Herman A., Weinraub Z., Soffer Y. & Caspi E. (1988) Ovarian hyperstimulation syndrome following D-Trp-6 luteinizing hormone releasing hormone microcapsules and menotropin for in vitro fertilization. *Fertility and Sterility* **50**, 912–916.

Goldberg G. L. & Runowicz C. D. (1992) Ovarian carcinoma of low malignant potential, infertility, and induction of ovulation-is there a link? *American Journal of Obstetrics and Gynecology* **166**, 853–854.

Homburg R., West C., Torresani T. & Jacobs H. S. (1990) Cotreatment with human growth hormone and gonadotrophins for induction of ovulation: a controlled clinical trial. *Fertility and Sterility* **53**, 254–260.

Howles C. (1990) GnRH analogues, past present and future uses in superovulation regimes. In: *Clinical IVF Forum*. (P. L. Matson, B. A. Lieberman, eds), Manchester University Press, Manchester, pp. 41–62.

Howles C., Macnamee M. C. & Edwards R. G. (1987) Short-term use of LHRH agonist to treat poor responders entering an in vitro fertilization (IVF) programme. *Human Reproduction* **2**, 655–656.

Howles C., Macnamee M. C., Edwards R. G., Goswamy R. & Steptoe P. C. (1986) Effect of high tonic levels of luteinizing hormone on outcome of in vitro fertilization. *Lancet* **2**, 521–522.

Hughes E. G., Federkow D. M., Daya S., Sagle M. A., Van de Koppel P. & Collins J. A. (1992) The routine use of gonadotropin-releasing hormone agonists prior to in vitro fertilization and gamete intrafallopian transfer: a meta-analysis of randomised controlled trials. *Fertility and Sterility* **58**, 888–896.

Jones H. W. Jr, Acosta A. A., Andrews M. C., Garcia J. E., Jones G. S., Mantzavinos T., McDowell J., Sandow B., Veeck L., Whibley Y., Wilkes C. & Wright G. (1983) The importance of the follicular phase to success and failure in in vitro fertilization. *Fertility and Sterility* **40**, 317–321.

Jones G. S., Acosta A. A., Garcia J. E., Bernardus R. E. & Rosenwaks Z. (1985) The effect of follicle-stimulating hormone without additional luteinizing hormone on follicular stimulation and oocyte development in normal ovulatory women. *Fertility and Sterility* **43**, 696–702.

Jones H. W. J. Jr., Jones G. S., Andrews M. C., Acosta A., Bundren C., Garcia J., Sandow B., Veeck L., Wilkes C., Witmyer J., Wortham J. E. & Wright G. (1982) The program for in vitro fertilization at Norfolk. *Fertility and Sterility* **38**, 14–21.

Katz E. (1993) The use of growth hormone treatment for ovulation induction. *Current Opinion in Obstetrics and Gynecology* **5**, 234–239.

Kempers R. D. (1994) Where are we going? *Fertility and Sterility* **62**, 686–689.

Knobil E. (1980) Neuroendocrine control of the menstrual cycle. *Recent Progress in Hormone Research* **36**, 53–88.

Lopata A. (1983) Concepts in human in vitro fertilization and embryo transfer. *Fertility and Sterility* **40**, 289–301.

Lunenfeld B. & Insler V. (1990) Induction of ovulation: historical aspects. *Bailliere's Clinical Obstetrics and Gynaecology* **4**, 473–489.

MacLachlan V., Besanko M., O'Shea F., Wade H., Wood C., Trounson A. & Healy D. L. (1989) A controlled study of luteinizing hormone-releasing hormone agonist (buserelin) for the induction of folliculogenesis before in vitro fertilization. *New England Journal of Medicine* **320,** 1233–1237.

Mannaerts B., de Leeuw R., Geelen J., Van Ravestein A., Van Wezenbeek P., Schuurs A. & Kloosterboer H. (1991) Comparative in vitro and in vivo studies on the biological characteristics of recombinant human follicle-stimulating hormone. *Endocrinology* **129,** 2623–2630.

Mannaerts B., Shoham Z., Schoot D., Bouchard P., Harlin J., Fauser B., Jacobs H., Rombout F. & Coelingh Bennink H. (1993) Single-dose pharmacokinetics and pharmacodynamics of recombinant human follicle-stimulating hormone (Org 32489) in gonadotropin-deficient volunteers. *Fertility and Sterility* **59,** 108–114.

Marrs R. P., Vargyas J. M., Gibbons W. E., Saito H. & Mishell D. R. Jr. (1983) A modified technique of human in vitro fertilization and embryo transfer. *American Journal of Obstetrics and Gynecology* **147,** 318–322.

Marrs R. P., Vargyas J. M., Shangold G. M. & Yee B. (1984) The effect of time of initiation of clomiphene citrate on multiple follicular development for human in vitro fertilization and embryo replacement procedures. *Fertility and Sterility* **41,** 682–685.

Medical Research International Society For Assisted Reproductive Technology, The American Fertility Society (1991) In Vitro fertilization and embryo transfer (IVF-ET) in the United States: 1989 results from the IVF-ET registry. *Fertility and Sterility* **55,** 14–23.

Medical Research International Society For Assisted Reproductive Technology, The American Fertility Society (1992) In Vitro fertilization and embryo transfer (IVF-ET) in the United States: 1990 results from the IVF-ET registry. *Fertility and Sterility* **57,** 15–24.

Meldrum D. R., Wiscot A., Hamilton F., Gutlay A. L., Huynh D. & Kempton W. (1988) Timing of initiation and dose schedule of leuprolide influence the time course of ovarian suppression. *Fertility and Sterility* **50,** 400–402.

Neveu S., Hedon B., Bringer J., Chinchole J. M., Arnal F., Humeau C., Cristol P. & Viala J. L. (1987) Ovarian stimulation by a combination of gonadotropin-releasing hormone agonist and gonadotropins for in vitro fertilization. *Fertility and Sterility* **47,** 639–643.

Oehninger S., Brzyski R. G., Muasher S. J., Acosta A. A. & Jones G. S. (1989) In vitro fertilization and embryo transfer in patients with endometriosis: impact of gonadotropin hormone-releasing hormone agonist. *Human Reproduction* **5,** 541.

Oehninger S., Toner J. P., Veeck L. L., Brzyski R. G., Acosta A. A. & Muasher S. J. (1992) Performance of cryopreserved pre-embryos obtained in in vitro fertilization cycles with or without a gonadotropin-releasing hormone agonist. *Fertility and Sterility* **57,** 620–625.

Owen E. J., Davies M. C., Kingsland C. R., Jacobs H. S. & Mason B. A. (1989) The use of a short regimen of buserelin, a gonadotrophin-releasing hormone agonist and human menopausal gonadotrophin in assisted conception cycles. *Human Reproduction* **4,** 749.

Porter R., Smith W., Craft I. L., Abdulwahid N. & Jacobs H. S. (1984) Induction of ovulation for in vitro fertilisation using buserelin and gonadotrophins. *Lancet* **2,** 1284–1285.

Quigley M. M., Collins R. L. & Blankstein J. (1988) Pure follicle stimulating hormone does not enhance follicular recruitment in clomiphene citrate/gonadotropin combinations. *Fertility and Sterility* **50,** 562–566.

Remohi J. & Pellicer A. (1993) Use of GnRH analogs in IVF. In: *Annual Progress in Reproductive Medicine: 1993*. (R. H. Asch, J. W. W. Studd, eds), Parthenon Publishing Group, Canforth, pp. 107–125.

Ron-El R., Golan A., Herman A., Nachum H., Soffer Y. & Caspi E. (1993) Assisted reproductive technologies. In: *Infertility: Male and Female*. (V. Insler, B. Lunenfeld, eds), second edition, Churchill Livingstone, London, pp. 525–562.

Ron-El R., Herman A., Golan A., Raziel A., Soffer Y. & Caspi E. (1989) Follicle cyst formation following long-acting gonadotropin-releasing hormone analog administration. *Fertility and Sterility* **52**, 1063–1066.

Salat-Baroux J., Alvarez S. & Antoine J. M. (1988) Results of IVF in the treatment of polycystic ovary disease. *Human Reproduction* **3**, 331.

Sampaio M., Serra V., Miro F., Calatayud C., Castellvi R. M. & Pellicer A. (1991) Development of ovarian cysts during gonadotrophin-releasing hormone agonists (GnRHa) administration. *Human Reproduction* **6**, 738–740.

Sassoon S. (1993) Ovulation induction agents and ovarian cancer. *Human Reproduction* **8**, 2246–2247 (letter).

Scoccia B., Blumenthal P., Wagner C., Prins G., Scommegna A. & Marut E. L. (1987) Comparison of urinary human follicle-stimulating hormone and human menopausal gonadotropins for ovarian stimulation in an in vitro fertilization program. *Fertility and Sterility* **48**, 446–449.

Smith W., Porter R., Ahuja K. & Craft I. L. (1984) Ultrasonic assessment of endometrial changes in stimulating cycles in an IVF and embryo transfer programme. *Journal of In Vitro Fertilization and Embryo Transfer* **1**, 233.

Stanger J. & Yovich J. L. (1985) Reduced in vitro fertilization of human oocytes from patients with raised basal luteinizing hormone levels during the follicular phase. *British Journal of Obstetrics and Gynaecology* **92**, 385–393.

Steptoe P. C. & Edwards R. G. (1978) Birth after the reimplantation of a human embryo. *Lancet* **2**, 336 (letter).

Tan S. L. (1994) Luteinizing hormone-releasing hormone agonists for ovarian stimulation in assisted reproduction. *Current Opinion in Obstetrics and Gynecology* **6**, 166–172.

Taubert H.-D. & Kuhl H. (1994) Steroids and steroid-like compounds. In: *Infertility: Male and Female*. (V. Insler, B. Lunenfeld, eds), second edition, Churchill Livingstone, Edinburgh, pp. 435–480.

Taymor M. L., Seibel M. M., Oskowitz S. P., Smith D. M. & Lee G. (1985) In Vitro fertilization and embryo transfer: an individualized approach to ovulation induction. *Journal of In Vitro Fertilization and Embryo Transfer* **2**, 162.

Trounson O. A., Leeton J. E., Wood C., Webb J. & Wood J. (1981) Pregnancies in human by fertilization in vitro and embryo transfer in the controlled ovulatory cycle. *Science* **212**, 681–682.

Tsirigotis M., Hutchon S., Yazdani N. & Craft I. (1995) The value of oestradiol estimations in controlled ovarian hyperstimulation cycles. *Human Reproduction* **10**, 972–973 (letter).

Van Uem J. F. H. M. & Hodgen G. D. (1986) Follicular growth, ovulation and the use of ovarian stimulants. In: *In Vitro Fertilisation; Past, Present, Future*. (S. Fishel, E. M. Symonds, eds), IRL Press, Oxford, pp. 27–42.

Volpe A., Coukos G., Artini P. G., Silferi M., Petralgia F., Boghen M., D'Ambrogio G. D. & Genazzani A. R. (1990) Pregnancy following combined growth hormone-pulsatile GnRH treatment in a patient with hypothalamic amenorrhoea. *Human Reproduction* **13**, 345–347.

Walker G. (1993) Profasi. In: *ABPI Data Sheet Compendium: 1993–94,* William Clowes Ltd, London, p.1521.

Whittemore A. S. (1993) Fertility drugs and the risk of ovarian cancer. *Human Reproduction* **8,** 999–1000.

Whittemore A. S., Harris R. & Intyre J. Collaborative Ovarian Cancer Group (1992) Characteristics relating to ovarian cancer risk: collaborative analysis of twelve US case-control studies. 2. Invasive epithelial ovarian cancer in white women. *American Journal of Epidemiology* **136,** 1184–1203.

Willemsen W., Kruitwagen R., Bastiaans B., Hanselaar T. & Rolland R. (1993) Ovarian stimulation and granulosa-cell tumour. *Lancet* **341,** 986–988.

Zorn J. R., Boyer P. & Guichard A. (1987) Never on a Sunday: programming for IVF-ET and GIFT. *Lancet* **1,** 385–386.

# 6

# Controlled superovulation for intrauterine insemination

GODWIN I. MENIRU, MARINOS TSIRIGOTIS and
IAN L. CRAFT

## Introduction

The wide variation in the reported incidence of pregnancy following intrauterine insemination (IUI) is a reflection of the multiplicity of factors that exert significant influences on the efficacy of this assisted conception technique. One of such factors is the use or non-use of ovarian stimulants. Many studies have shown a significantly poorer outcome when IUI is carried out in a natural ovarian cycle instead of a stimulated cycle (Ombelet et al. 1995). Ovarian stimulation, by ensuring production of more than one oocyte, improves the chances of fertilisation and subsequent establishment of pregnancy in subfertile couples. It is also possible that ovarian stimulation corrects unsuspected ovulatory dysfunction (Arici et al. 1994) and luteal phase defects (Edwards & Brody 1995). Superovulation for IUI aims at the production of three and certainly not more than four mature fertilisable oocytes. Ovulation of a greater number of oocytes could lead to an unacceptably high incidence of higher order multiple pregnancies unless the treatment cycle is converted to an in vitro fertilisation (IVF) cycle or cancelled when excessive ovarian response is noted. Several methods of stimulation have been used for IUI and are shown in Table 6.1. It appears that the success of any particular regimen depends on the number of mature oocytes produced and not necessarily on the drug that is used (Ombelet et al. 1995). This chapter will deal with common protocols of ovarian stimulation for the purpose of IUI. Case summaries will be presented to illustrate the various regimens and associated patterns of patient response.

## Prediction of ovulation

The ability to accurately predict the time of ovulation is one of the most important determinants of success with IUI because it allows optimal timing of

Table 6.1. *Regimens for ovarian stimulation*

Natural cycle
CC
CC + hMG
CC + FSH
hMG
FSH
hMG + FSH
GnRHa + hMG
GnRHa + FSH
GnRHa + hMG + FSH

*Notes:*
CC: clomiphene citrate; FSH: follicle stimulating hormone: GnRHa: gonadotrophin releasing hormone agonist; hMG: human menopausal gonadotrophin.

insemination. This becomes even more crucial when thawed frozen semen is used because longevity of the spermatozoa is shortened. The use of basal body temperature measurement is inappropriate as diagnosis of ovulation is retrospective. Changes in cervical mucus are unreliable because the interval between appearance of the pre-ovulatory type of mucus and ovulation itself is highly variable. Moreover, induction of multiple follicular development with resulting supraphysiological plasma oestrogen concentration may confuse issues further by distorting the pattern of cervical mucus production. Ovarian ultrasound scanning and detection of the luteinising hormone (LH) surge are two methods that can be used to aid decision on when to carry out insemination. Each is capable of being used independently but their combined use improves the accuracy of monitoring. The more frequently these are carried out the greater the accuracy of the timing but this will be at the expense of patient comfort and would entail increased costs.

A major goal of ultrasound scanning during the period of follicular stimulation is to exact the timing of human chorionic gonadotrophin (hCG) administration. Injection of hCG acts as a surrogate LH surge whose onset is known with certainty and can be used to accurately time the onset of ovulation. The aim is always to administer the injection before the endogenous surge of LH commences. On the other hand one should avoid premature administration of hCG as this will lead to suboptimal outcome of the treatment cycle. hCG is usually administered at a dose of 10000 IU when the leading follicles reach a diameter of 18 mm or more. Administration of the injection in an IUI treatment cycle is however conditional on not more than four follicles (preferably three), measuring 16 mm and above, being present. hCG is also withheld if eight or more follicles with diameters above 12 mm are seen (Edwards & Brody 1995). The endogenous LH surge will not be detected in programmes where only ultrasound monitoring is carried out and it may occur before the follicles have reached the required size for hCG administration. Up to 20% of patients treated with clomiphene citrate and human menopausal gonadotrophin (hMG) will exhibit this phenomenon before the leading follicles reach 18–20 mm in diameter (Macnamee *et al.* 1988). Experience from IVF cycles suggests that if the surge is detected and hCG administered immediately, the patient's performance in that cycle will not be compromised (Macnamee & Brinsden 1992). The utility of this manoeuvre in IUI is not yet clear although similar conclusions may be applicable.

Patients are encouraged to purchase home LH test kits and carry out the test on the first urine sample of the day. As these ovulation prediction kits are relatively expensive it is important to limit, as much as possible, the period of usage. One way of estimating when to do the tests is to study the woman's menstrual history and determine the average day of ovulation. She is then instructed to start the tests from 4 days before that day. For example, with a history of a 28-day menstrual cycle, the LH monitoring tests are commenced on day 11 of the stimulation cycle. If the menstrual history is not helpful, the tests are started as soon as the leading follicle reaches 16 mm in diameter.

### Timing of insemination

Two inseminations are performed 24 and 48 hours, respectively, from the time of hCG administration. The expectation is that viable spermatozoa will be present in the female genital tract at the time of ovulation. The issue of optimal number of inseminations has not been resolved; contradictory findings have been reported in the literature for both husband and donor sperm (Centola *et al.* 1990; Silverberg *et al.* 1992; Ransom *et al.* 1994; Khalifa *et al.* 1995; Ombelet *et al.* 1995). Resolution of two key uncertainties may help resolve this controversy. Firstly, it is not known how long the oocyte remains fertilisable in vivo following ovulation. Experience from in vitro studies suggest that fertilisation of the oocyte is still possible 24 hours or more after ovulation, contrary to the previous traditional teaching of 12 hours. Secondly, the period of survival and retention of fertilising ability of the inseminated spermatozoa is uncertain. Spermatozoa may retain their fertilising capacity for many days under favourable culture conditions but artefacts resulting from sperm preparation techniques and the freeze-thaw process may impede viability and longevity of the

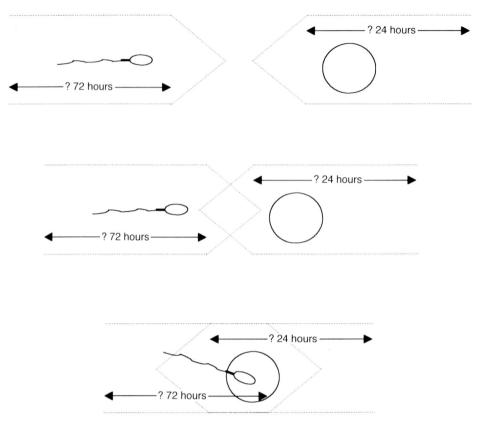

Figure 6.1. Coordination of insemination and ovulation: pivotal role of the period of gamete viability.

respective sperm populations. Cycle monitoring, administration of hCG and insemination should allow satisfactory overlap of the period of viability of the inseminated spermatozoa and ovulated oocytes (Figure 6.1). Oocyte release after hCG injection occurs in waves and not all at once (Abbasi *et al.* 1987). Therefore the second insemination that is carried out 48 hours after hCG injection is still appropriate, given that not all oocytes will be released 37 hours after that injection. Pelvic ultrasound scanning is performed at the second insemination to confirm ovulation. Follicular rupture and the presence of free fluid in the pouch of Douglas are features that support this diagnosis. A moot question is what to do if at that scanning episode the follicles have not ruptured. One option will be to schedule a third insemination 24 hours later but the utility of this is not clear at present. Follicular rupture may occur before then in which case, spermatozoa delivered by either the second insemination or both of the previous two inseminations may fertilise the released oocytes. If the LH surge is detected a decision has to be made regarding whether to administer hCG or not. Either way, a single insemination is carried out as soon as possible that same day. Alternatively two inseminations are carried out; the first being on the day the LH surge is detected while the second insemination is performed 24 hours later.

### Natural cycle

Insemination in a natural cycle is performed once or twice as detailed above following detection of the LH surge. There is usually no need for intensive ultrasound monitoring; the first scan can be performed on day 9 and subsequent scans planned accordingly. The most important monitoring method here is that of LH surge detection. This surge appears to commence between midnight and 08.00 hours in a large proportion of cases (Lenton 1993). It follows that testing a first morning urine sample will detect any surge commencing during the preceding night. Insemination is performed on the day of LH surge detection and optionally repeated 24 hours later.

### Clomiphene citrate

This drug is administered at a dose of 100 mg from days 2 to 6. The dose of clomiphene citrate may be increased to 150 mg but it is more appropriate to consider other stimulation protocols rather than further increasing the dose to 200 mg or more. Monitoring is commenced on day 9 with ultrasound scanning. hCG may be administered or a spontaneous LH surge awaited. In each instance, data on outcome of treatment should be accumulated and analysed at intervals in order to find out which option is more effective.

### Clomiphene citrate and gonadotrophins

The combination of clomiphene citrate and exogenous gonadotrophin administration achieves a balance between efficacy and cost. Clomiphene citrate is administered together with hMG or follicle stimulating hormone (FSH) preparations. The growth of ovarian follicles, recruited as a result of the clomiphene citrate-induced increase in endogenous production of FSH, is maintained by subsequent hMG or FSH injections. Following onset of a natural menstrual period or withdrawal bleeding, clomiphene citrate is administered orally from days 2 to 6 at the dose of 100 mg daily (Figure 6.2). hMG or FSH is administered as a single intramuscular injection at the dose of 150 IU on days 5 and 7. The patient then has her first ultrasound scan on day 9 to ascertain the number and size of ovarian follicles as well as to measure the

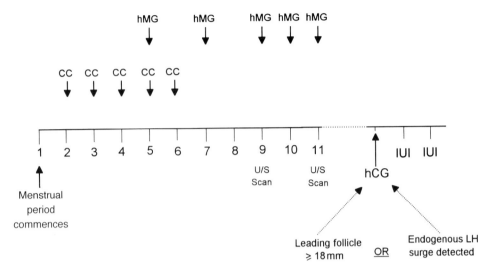

Figure 6.2. The clomiphene citrate (CC)/gonadotrophin stimulation regimen. hMG: human menopausal gonadotrophin; hCG: human chorionic gonadotrophin; IUI: intrauterine insemination; LH: luteinising hormone; U/S: ultrasound.

thickness of the endometrium. Administration of gonadotrophins is then continued at a dose of 75–150 IU daily or on alternate days, until the leading follicle measures 18 mm or more and endometrial thickness is at least 8.5 mm (usually above 10 mm) and of grade 'A' quality (see Chapter 7). While the dose of clomiphene citrate is fixed at 100 mg, the dose of gonadotrophins varies depending on factors such as the patient's history, response to ovarian stimulation, anthropometric indices or similar measures of obesity, age and polycystic appearance of the ovaries.

### Gonadotrophins

hMG, FSH or rarely a combination of both, can be administered on alternate days starting from day 3. The dose to be administered on each occasion is individualised but 150 IU is usually average. This is adjusted following the first ultrasound scan which is carried out on day 9. It is also decided at this time whether to continue on the alternate day regimen or change to daily injections. Many workers have also used a daily injection regimen starting from day 2 or 3 of the treatment cycle and continuing till the time of hCG administration or spontaneous LH surge.

### Agonist and gonadotrophins

Problems with cycle control in relation to the LH surge may lead to consideration of drug regimens incorporating gonadotrophin releasing hormone agonists (GnRHa). The increased costs from the use of the agonist, the increased utilisation of exogenous gonadotrophins as well as the need for progesterone supplementation in the luteal phase and first trimester of any resulting pregnancy, may make this option unattractive to some. On the other hand, cycles conducted without the benefit of GnRHa may incur increased costs due to the use of LH kits, more frequent ultrasound scanning, oestradiol and other hormone assays and cancelled cycles from premature LH surges. This may decrease or eliminate the price differential between GnRHa and non-GnRHa cycles. The full potentials of IUI cannot be exploited if factors that control its efficacy are not optimised. It is generally agreed that incorporation of GnRHa into ovarian stimulation regimens leads to a greater control of ovarian function allowing more flexibility to the scheduling of hCG injections and subsequent activities. For example, hCG administration may be withheld until the desired follicle number and size are achieved, without fear of an endogenous surge of LH. Insemination can be scheduled to take place during predetermined days in the week as is presently the case for IVF in many units. Patients and staff will also find this more convenient.

The short protocols may be initially attractive options for ovarian stimulation in IUI treatment cycles but in a recent report (Chung *et al.* 1995), it was suggested that the long protocol is a better method. This is because the 'flare-up' effect present in the first few days of GnRHa administration may elicit abnormal plasma hormonal concentrations during the period of follicular stimulation which usually commences within a day or two in the short protocols. These transient elevations of hormone levels are not present when full downregulation has taken place as is the norm in the long protocol. Ovarian stimulation is started with daily injections of 150 IU of hMG and/or FSH from day 1, 2 or 3 of the treatment cycles (short protocols) or after 2 weeks of daily or depot GnRHa administration. The dose is subsequently readjusted depending on the patient's response. hCG is administered when the usual criteria are met.

## Case summaries

### Case 1

This patient insisted on having IUI performed in a natural ovarian cycle and she had reasonably regular menstrual periods. Her first ultrasound scan on day 9 showed a dominant ovarian follicle measuring 15 mm in diameter. She was asked to commence urinary LH testing and the test became positive on day 13. IUI was performed that same day and repeated 24 hours later by which time ultrasound scanning showed features compatible with ovulation (Figure 6.3).

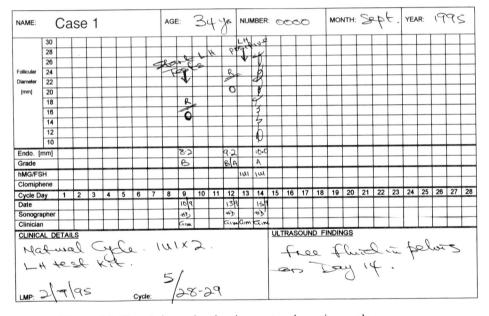

Figure 6.3. Case 1: insemination in a natural ovarian cycle.

## Case 2

Following a 5 day course of clomiphene citrate three follicles were visualised during ultrasound scanning on day 9. Daily urinary dipstick testing for the LH surge was commenced the following day as one of the follicles measured 16 mm in diameter. hCG was administered on day 12 when that follicle measured 20 mm and IUI was performed 24 and 48 hours later (Figure 6.4).

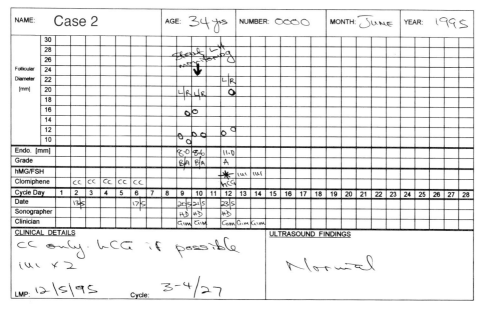

Figure 6.4. Case 2: the use of clomiphene citrate for ovarian stimulation.

## Case 3

A combination of clomiphene citrate and hMG was utilised for ovarian stimulation here. Although seven follicles were seen at the initial scan only five were noted on day 13 and three of them measured 18 mm and above. LH surge detection tests were not performed in this cycle (Figure 6.5).

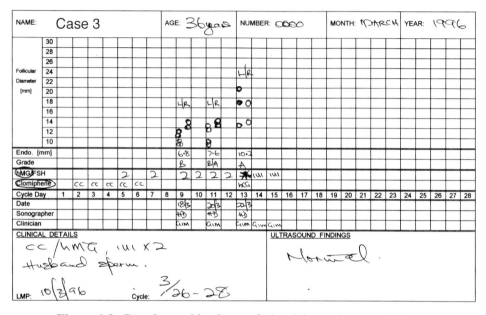

Figure 6.5. Case 3: combined use of clomiphene citrate and human menopausal gonadotrophin.

## Case 4

This case illustrates the use of clomiphene citrate and FSH for controlled superovulation. Only two episodes of ultrasound scanning were required. Testing for the LH surge was commenced on day 11 in view of the patient's menstrual cycle length. It will be noted that one of the follicles had reached a diameter of 16 mm on day 9 (Figure 6.6).

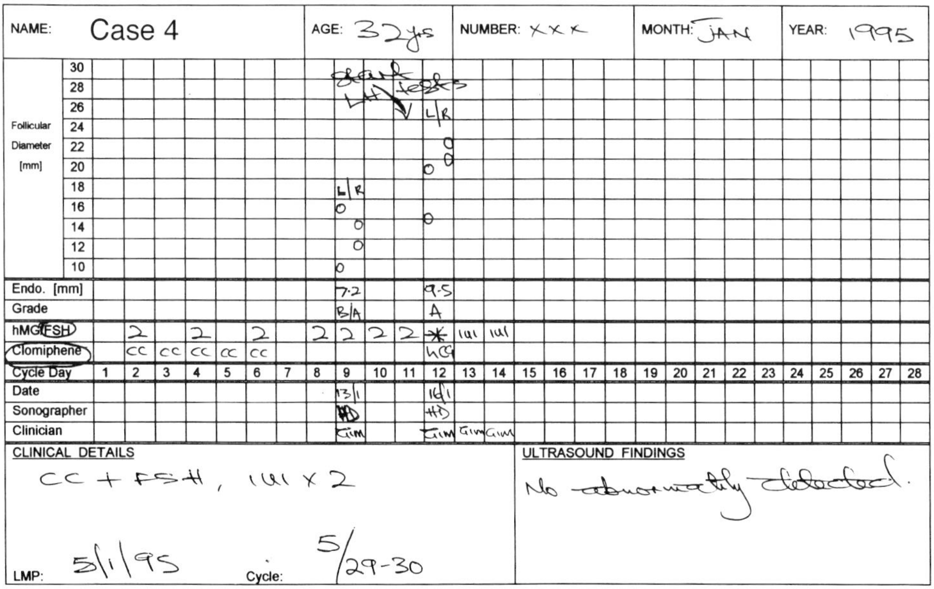

Figure 6.6. Case 4: use of clomiphene citrate and follicle stimulating hormone injections for superovulation.

## Case 5

Alternate day administration of hMG until day 8 resulted in the development of six follicles. Daily injections were commenced from day 9 to stimulate further growth of the follicles. Three of these follicles reached the required diameter at the last scanning episode before administration of hCG (Figure 6.7).

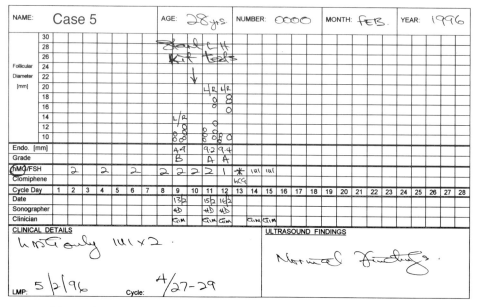

Figure 6.7. Case 5: sole use of human menopausal gonadotrophin for ovarian stimulation.

## Case 6

The short protocol of buserelin administration with FSH injections is illustrated here (Figure 6.8). An initial ultrasound scan was required on day 3 to exclude ovarian pathology. Although three follicles were recruited by the FSH injections, their growth was not satisfactory on day 9, so the dose of FSH was increased for a few days. The long interval between the last two scanning episodes in the treatment cycle shows one of the benefits of abolishing the endogenous LH surge with agonists.

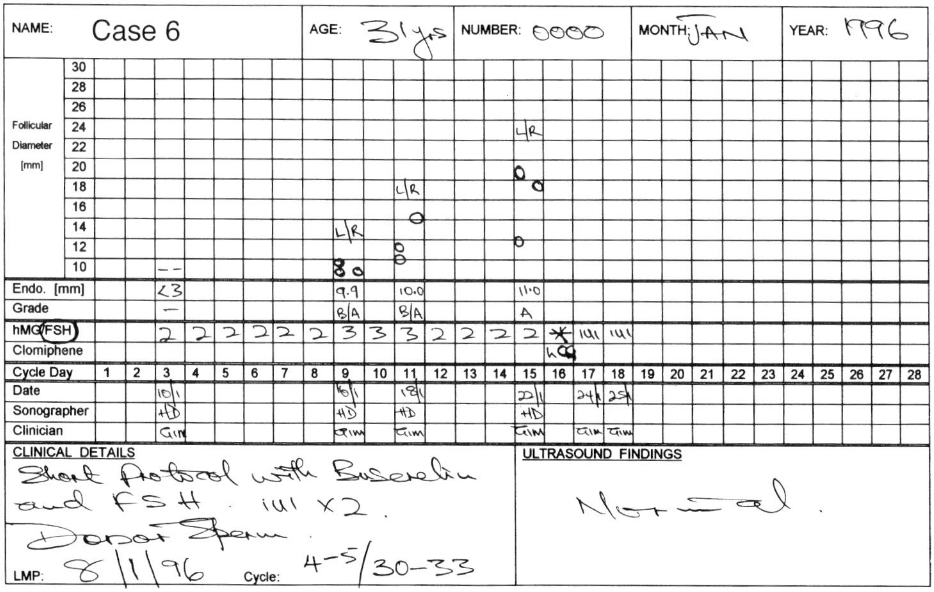

Figure 6.8. Case 6: the short protocol of buserelin administration for intrauterine insemination.

## Case 7

This 42-year-old woman wanted to try for a pregnancy with her own oocytes despite patient information on the age-related decline in fecundity that operates through oocyte quality. The first IVF cycle conducted with the long protocol was converted to an IUI cycle due to the development of very few follicles (Figure 6.9). The protocol of buserelin administration was changed to the short type in the second attempt at IVF but her response was still poor and timed sexual intercourse (TSI) was advised (Figure 6.10).

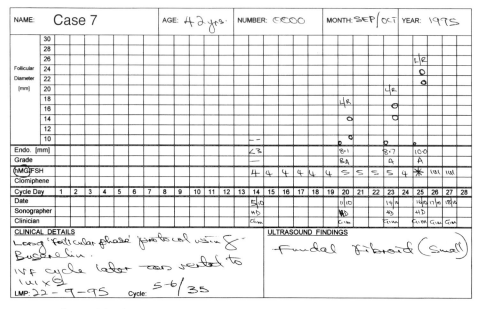

Figure 6.9. Case 7: conversion of an in vitro fertilisation cycle to an intrauterine insemination cycle.

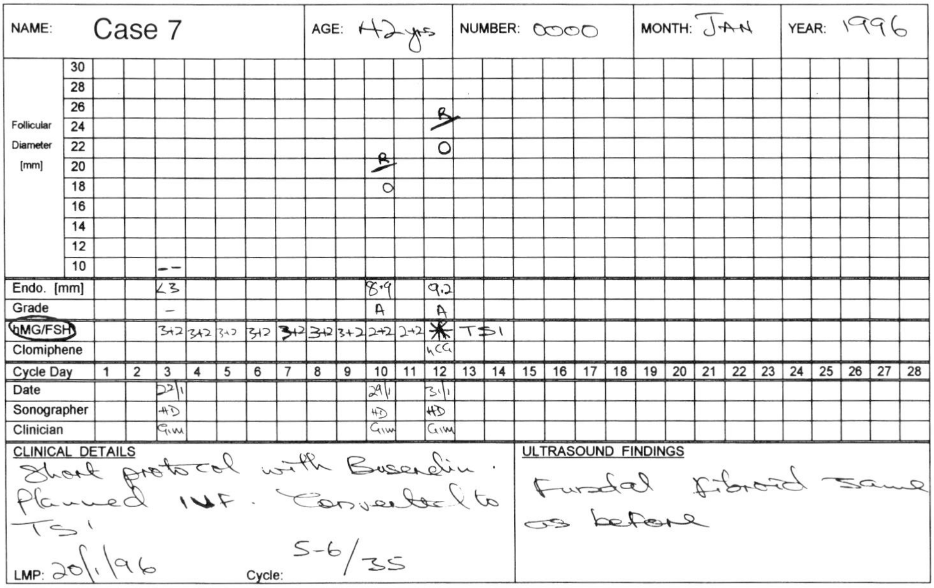

NAME: Case 7 | AGE: 42yrs | NUMBER: 0000 | MONTH: JAN | YEAR: 1996

| | | | | | | | | | | | | | | | | | | | | | | | | | | | | |
|---|---|---|---|---|---|---|---|---|---|---|---|---|---|---|---|---|---|---|---|---|---|---|---|---|---|---|---|---|
| Follicular Diameter [mm] | | | | | | | | | | | | | | | | | | | | | | | | | | | | |
| 30 | | | | | | | | | | | | | | | | | | | | | | | | | | | | |
| 28 | | | | | | | | | | | | | | | | | | | | | | | | | | | | |
| 26 | | | | | | | | | | | | | | | | | | | | | | | | | | | | |
| 24 | | | | | | | | | | | | R | | | | | | | | | | | | | | | | |
| 22 | | | | | | | | | | | | O | | | | | | | | | | | | | | | | |
| 20 | | | | | | | | | | R | | | | | | | | | | | | | | | | | | |
| 18 | | | | | | | | | | O | | | | | | | | | | | | | | | | | | |
| 16 | | | | | | | | | | | | | | | | | | | | | | | | | | | | |
| 14 | | | | | | | | | | | | | | | | | | | | | | | | | | | | |
| 12 | | | | | | | | | | | | | | | | | | | | | | | | | | | | |
| 10 | | | -- | | | | | | | | | | | | | | | | | | | | | | | | | |
| Endo. [mm] | | | <3 | | | | | | | 8.9 | | 9.2 | | | | | | | | | | | | | | | | |
| Grade | | | – | | | | | | | A | | A | | | | | | | | | | | | | | | | |
| hMG/FSH | | | 3+2 | 3+2 | 3+2 | 3+2 | 3+2 | 3+2 | 3+2 | 2+2 | 2+2 | * | TSI | | | | | | | | | | | | | | | |
| Clomiphene | | | | | | | | | | | | hCG | | | | | | | | | | | | | | | | |
| Cycle Day | 1 | 2 | 3 | 4 | 5 | 6 | 7 | 8 | 9 | 10 | 11 | 12 | 13 | 14 | 15 | 16 | 17 | 18 | 19 | 20 | 21 | 22 | 23 | 24 | 25 | 26 | 27 | 28 |
| Date | | | 22/1 | | | | | | | 29/1 | | 31/1 | | | | | | | | | | | | | | | | |
| Sonographer | | | HD | | | | | | | HD | | HD | | | | | | | | | | | | | | | | |
| Clinician | | | GM | | | | | | | GM | | GM | | | | | | | | | | | | | | | | |

CLINICAL DETAILS

Short protocol with Buserelin. Planned IVF. Converted to TSI

LMP: 20/1/96 Cycle: 5-6/35

ULTRASOUND FINDINGS

Fundal fibroid same as before

Figure 6.10. Case 7: conversion of an in vitro fertilisation cycle to 'timed sexual intercourse'.

## Case 8

Problems encountered during superovulation in females with polycystic ovaries are shown in Figures 6.11–6.13. A first IUI cycle using clomiphene citrate and FSH was cancelled due to poor response. The second cycle was also cancelled, because of over-response to the increased dose of FSH that was used. Repeat of the clomiphene citrate/FSH regimen in the third cycle produced a more acceptable response pattern and insemination was performed following administration of hCG.

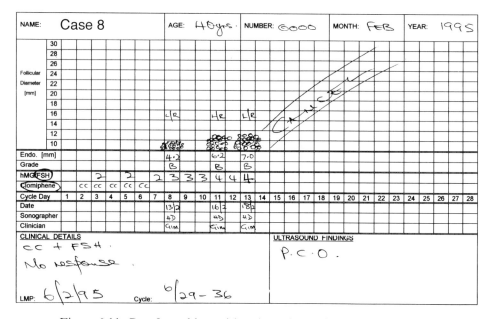

Figure 6.11. Case 8: problem with polycystic ovaries: cancellation of cycle due to poor response.

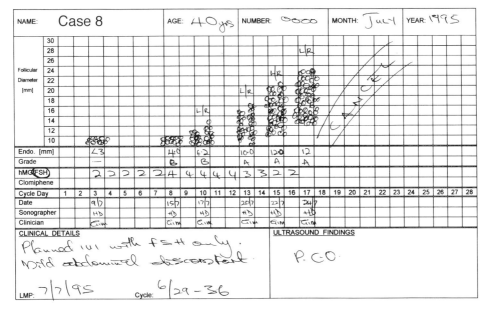

Figure 6.12. Case 8: problem with polycystic ovaries: cancellation of cycle from over-response.

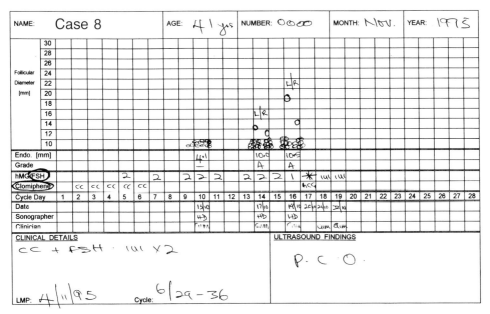

Figure 6.13. Case 8: problem with polycystic ovaries: an intrauterine insemination cycle that worked!

## Case 9

Over-response in this case was managed by converting the treatment cycle from IUI to IVF (Figure 6.14). This patient also had polycystic ovaries. She later on manifested features of moderate ovarian hyperstimulation syndrome.

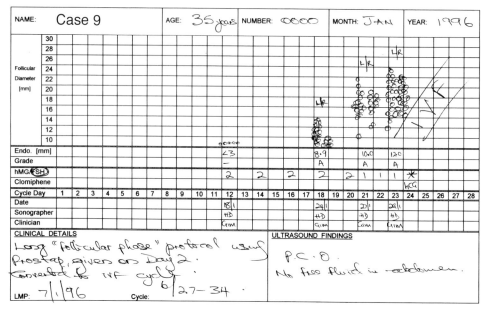

Figure 6.14. Case 9: problem with polycystic ovaries: conversion to an in vitro fertilisation cycle.

## Case 10

Some women may have intermittent vaginal bleeding during the period of ovarian stimulation. Our experience is that such women rarely get pregnant in that treatment cycle. We therefore discontinue superovulation in any treatment cycle where this bleeding is noted (Figure 6.15).

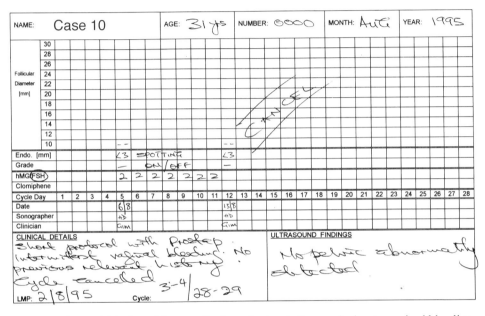

Figure 6.15. Case 10: cancellation of stimulation cycle due to vaginal bleeding.

## References

Abbasi R., Kenigsberg D., Danforth D., Falk R. J. & Hodgen G. D. (1987) Cumulative ovulation rate in human menopausal/human chorionic gonadotropin-treated monkeys: 'step-up' versus 'step-down' dose regimens. *Fertility and Sterility* **47**, 1019–1024.

Arici A., Byrd W., Bradshaw K., Kutteh W. H., Marshburn P. & Carr B. R. (1994) Evaluation of clomiphene citrate and human chorionic gonadotropin treatment: a prospective, randomized, crossover study during intrauterine insemination cycles. *Fertility and Sterility* **61**, 314–318.

Centola G. M., Mattox J. H. & Rauberts R. F. (1990) Pregnancy rates after double versus single insemination with frozen donor semen. *Fertility and Sterility* **54**, 1089–1092.

Chung C. C., Fleming R., Jamieson M. E., Yates R. W. S. & Coutts J. R. T. (1995) Randomized comparison of ovulation induction with or without intrauterine insemination in the treatment of unexplained infertility. *Human Reproduction* **10**, 3139–3141.

Edwards R. G. & Brody S. A. (1995) Natural cycle and ovarian stimulation in assisted conception. In: *Principles and Practice of Assisted Human Reproduction.* W. B. Saunders Company, Philadelphia, pp. 233–284.

Khalifa Y., Redgement C. J., Tsirigotis M., Grudzinskas J. G. & Craft I. L. (1995) The value of single versus repeated insemination in intra-uterine donor insemination cycles. *Human Reproduction* **10,** 153–154.

Lenton E. A. (1993) Ovulation timing. In: *Donor Insemination.* (C. L. R. Barratt, I. D. Cooke, eds), Cambridge University Press, Cambridge, pp. 97–110.

Macnamee M. C. & Brinsden P. R. (1992) Superovulation strategies in assisted conception. In: *A Textbook of In Vitro Fertilization and Assisted Reproduction.* (P. R. Brinsden & P. A. Rainsbury, eds), Parthenon Publishing Group, Carnforth, pp. 111–125.

Macnamee M. C., Edwards R. G. & Howles C. M. (1988) The influence of stimulation regimes and luteal phase support on the outcome of IVF. *Human Reproduction* **3** (supplement 2), 43–52.

Ombelet W., Puttemans P. & Bosmans E. (1995) Intrauterine insemination: a first-step procedure in the algorithm of male subfertility treatment. *Human Reproduction* **10** (supplement 1), 90–102.

Ransom M. X., Blotner M. B., Bohrer M., Corsan G. & Kemmann E. (1994) Does increasing frequency of intrauterine insemination improve pregnancy rates significantly during superovulation cycles? *Fertility and Sterility* **61,** 303–307.

Silverberg K. M., Johnson J. V., Olive D. L., Burns W. N. & Schenken R. S. (1992) A prospective, randomized trial comparing two different intrauterine insemination regimens in controlled ovarian hyperstimulation cycles. *Fertility and Sterility* **57,** 357–361.

# 7
# Ultrasonography in the management of infertility with special reference to intrauterine insemination

GODWIN I. MENIRU and IAN L. CRAFT

### Introduction

Reports on the use of ultrasonography for visualising the pelvic organs and studying ovarian follicular changes first appeared in the scientific literature of the 1970s (Kratochowil *et al.* 1972; Hackeloer 1977). Initially, transabdominal ultrasound scanning only was used. Although still currently in use this technique suffers from the drawback of requiring a distended bladder, which can be very uncomfortable for the patient, particularly when pressure is applied on the lower abdomen during scanning. It is not uncommon for patients to wait for a while after arrival at the unit, drinking large volumes of fluid, in order for the bladder to fill and become distended. Furthermore, accurate delineation of pelvic structures may not be possible in some women due to beam scatter by excessive subcutaneous fat or scars from previous operations (Tan *et al.* 1992) or overlying gas-filled bowel loops. Transabdominal scanning utilises frequencies of between 2.5 and 3.5 MHz. Introduction of the transvaginal transducer has done away with the inconvenience of having a full bladder for this procedure as well as allowing for a more detailed visualisation of the uterus, ovary and other pelvic structures. In fact having a full bladder may make transvaginal scanning more difficult because the distended bladder displaces pelvic organs and tissue further away from the vaginally placed transducer. In some cases however, a full bladder may be required to straighten out an acutely anteverted uterus in order to improve its visualisation (Figure 7.1). Transvaginal sonography is particularly useful when there is a retroverted uterus. Higher ultrasound frequencies (5–7.5 MHz) can be used thereby improving the resolution of the image but the structures have to be within 6 cm of the transducer for optimal imaging at these frequencies. Structures beyond 8–9 cm may not be imaged transvaginally (Fried 1995) and the use of both scanning routes is often needed for complete evaluation of large pelvic masses.

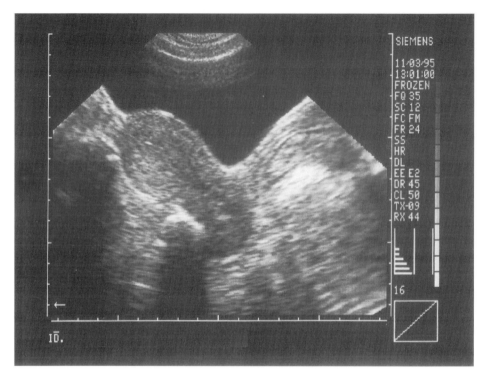

Figure 7.1. Transabdominal sonogram: anteverted uterus and distended bladder.

To reduce the risk of cross infection the vaginal transducer is covered with a disposable condom. A water-based ultrasound gel is placed on the inside surface of the condom tip before pulling it over the transducer. This gel acts as an acoustic couplant by obliterating the air interface between the transducer head and the condom material, further improving the image obtained during scanning. The probe itself is washed at regular intervals during the day, or at least at the end of each working day, with antiseptic solution and rinsed thoroughly. Ultrasonography has profoundly influenced medical practice in recent years and this is more so in infertility management where it has both diagnostic and therapeutic uses. It is difficult imagining the conduct of modern day assisted conception treatment without the use of the ultrasound scanner. This chapter will deal with the applicability of ultrasonography to the management of infertility with special reference to intrauterine insemination (IUI). It does not aim to teach the technique of ultrasound scanning. Rather, it is an account of features that the practitioner will frequently come across or hear mentioned during activities related to the management of infertile women and IUI. Relevant pelvic pathologies which are amenable to sonographic diagnosis will also be described. Other indications and benefits of this monitoring tool in the sphere of infertility management will be mentioned at the conclusion of the chapter.

## Diagnosis of pelvic pathology

Ultrasound scanning provides useful information relating to the presence or absence of pelvic pathology and is optimally carried out before commencement of assisted conception treatment. Using ultrasound scanning in this way complements information derived from the patient's clinical history, physical examination and other investigations. The timing of this evaluative scan is not universally agreed but it could be scheduled for the early follicular phase of the menstrual cycle. The importance of this scan cannot be overemphasised. Previously undiagnosed pelvic pathology may be discovered which could contraindicate IUI (e.g. tubal or endometrial pathology) or lead to a modification of the stimulation protocol (e.g. polycystic ovaries). The scanning technique depends on particular circumstances and size of the pelvic organs and tumours. Transabdominal scanning, for example, will yield more information when there are pelvic enlargements of more than 5 cm (Fleischer & Entman 1991a).

### *Müllerian duct developmental defects*

Varying degrees of failure of development, fusion or canalisation of the Müllerian ducts before birth may lead to characteristic defects (Figure 7.2). Some of these malformations have no impact on the fertility potential of the female while others may cause varying degrees of difficulty with achieving pregnancy. Oligomenorrhoea, menorrhagia and dysmenorrhoea are also presenting features in some cases, and obstruction to the outflow of menstrual blood loss occurs when there is failure of canalisation of any part of the female genital tract distal to the endometrial cavity. Although developmental defects of the Müllerian duct were originally thought to be uncommon, present day evidence suggests that they may be present in up to 2–3% of females (Sanfillippo *et al.* 1978, 1986). Furthermore it has been estimated that 25% of women with congenital uterine anomalies may have difficulty becoming pregnant (Abramovici *et al.* 1983; Ansbacher 1983; Golan *et al.* 1989). It is therefore important to carefully study the shape of the uterus during ultrasound scanning as this may offer the first clue to the existence of a malformation, especially in those who did not have hysterosalpingography or hysteroscopy prior to this. Adoption of a systematic scanning technique will prevent any malformation from being

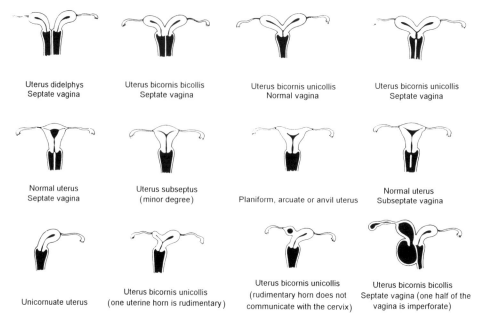

Figure 7.2. Müllerian duct defects. Adapted from Tindall (1987).

missed as well as ensuring that its exact configuration is determined (Figure 7.3). Any woman in whom an abnormality is detected should be evaluated further to determine whether that particular type is associated with infertility or a pregnancy-related problem. Known problems in pregnancy include recurrent miscarriage, premature delivery, malpresentation, intrauterine growth retardation and morbid adherence of the placenta. Corrective surgical treatment may be required in carefully selected cases before proceeding with attempts to aid conception. Finally it should be borne in mind that malformations of the genital tract tend to occur in conjunction with those of the urinary tract. Detailed scanning of the kidneys, ureters and bladder and other investigations of urinary tract function, should be carried out whenever Müllerian duct defects are found.

### *Uterine leiomyoma*

Uterine leiomyomata are common findings during pelvic ultrasound scanning. Up to 20% or more of females may harbour one or more of these benign smooth muscle tumours, and the incidence is high in those of African descent. Whenever they are found their size and position should be accurately determined. Details of the sonographic features of uterine leiomyoma can be found in Fleischer & Entman (1991a). Basically they appear as hypoechoic solid

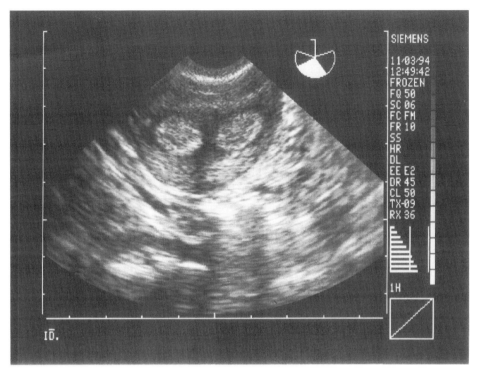

Figure 7.3. Transvaginal sonogram (transverse section): a bicornuate uterus. There are two distinct endometrial cavities separated by a central core of myometrium. A systematic scanning technique will allow identification of the exact type and level of malformation (see Figure 7.2).

masses within the uterus. Apart from 3% of leiomyomata that are of cervical origin, the rest are found in the fundus and corpus of the uterus (Fleischer & Entman 1991a). Although a single tumour may be found in some cases, the usual finding is for many tumours of varying sizes in the uterus. As they increase in size they compress adjacent myometrial fibres which subsequently form a false capsule around them. Some leiomyomata lie wholly in the myometrium (intramural type) while others project towards the peritoneal surface of the uterus (subserous type) or bulge into the uterine cavity (submucous type (Figures 7.4 and 7.5). The subserous or submucous types may ultimately become pedunculated. Most leiomyomata are asymptomatic and only discovered incidental to pelvic examination or ultrasound scanning in well-woman clinic settings. When symptomatic, presenting features include abnormal vaginal bleeding, an abdomino-pelvic mass and pain, the latter being more common in pregnancy. Habitual abortion is also a feature but this is likely to be uncommon and other aetiologies should first be excluded. The

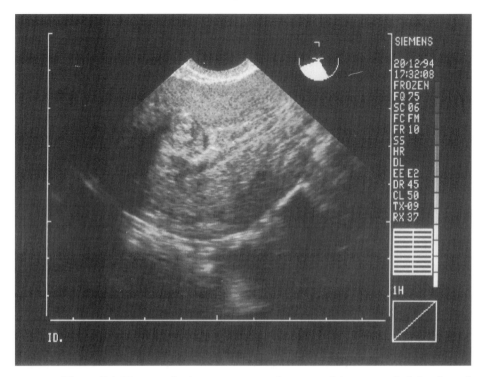

Figure 7.4. Transvaginal sonogram: a submucous leiomyoma bulging into the endometrial cavity from the anterior fundal aspect of the uterus.

relationship between uterine leiomyoma and infertility is nebulous and consequently controversial except in rare cases of bilateral cornual blockage. Antifertility effects are more likely in situations where the endometrial cavity is distorted by one or more of these tumours.

Great care has to be exercised in deciding which patients need treatment because there is a potential danger of further compromising the patient's fertility. An embarked myomectomy operation may end in a hysterectomy due to technical problems or complications. The risk of this happening increases in repeat operations carried out for recurrent uterine leiomyoma. There is a significant risk of adhesions forming after the operation although current techniques such as laparoscopic myomectomy, use of fibrin sealants or absorbable adhesion barriers (Interceed; Johnson & Johnson Medical Ltd, Ascot, UK) decreases the incidence and severity of this problem. The chance of pregnancy occurring after myomectomy does not seem to exceed 40% (Healy et al. 1986). Creation of a hypo-oestrogenic state with gonadotrophin releasing hormone agonists tends to lead to regression of these tumours but this effect is temporary unless myomectomy is then performed.

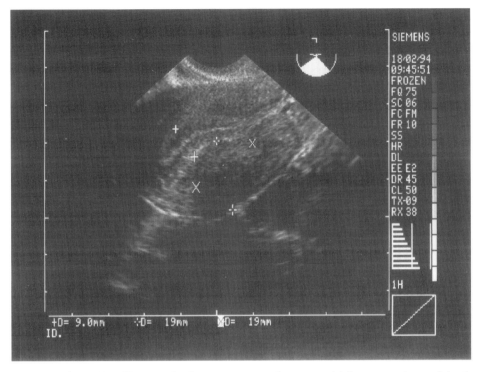

Figure 7.5. Transvaginal sonogram: an intramural leiomyoma located in the posterior wall of the uterus from where it is bulging towards the endometrium and indenting it.

## *Polyps and cervical pathology*

Polyps in the cervical and uterine canals may be incidental findings during ultrasound evaluation of the infertile woman (Figures 7.6 and 7.7) but their removal before further treatment is necessary, at least to confirm their benign nature if not to cure an associated abnormal vaginal bleeding. The importance of Nabothian follicles (Figures 7.8 and 7.9) derive mainly from the very uncommon situation where the presence of numerous cysts may give initial appearances similar to those of developing ovarian follicles. A good scanning technique, however, largely eliminates this problem especially in subsequent scans when the size of these cysts will be seen to be relatively stationary unlike that of the developing ovarian follicles.

## *Endometriosis and endometriomas*

Sonographic diagnosis of endometriosis relies on a highly suggestive clinical history and findings on pelvic examination as there does not seem to be a

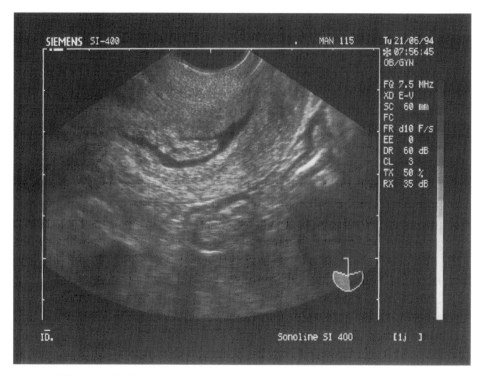

Figure 7.6. Transvaginal sonogram: a cervical polyp clearly demonstrated because of distension of the cervical canal by mucus.

characteristic ultrasonic feature. Endometriotic lesions appear cystic, solid or mixed on ultrasound scanning. In other cases no definite sonographic lesion exists as the endometriotic process often leads to fibrosis of affected tissues and not the formation of masses. Blumenfeld *et al.* (1990) described various features of endometriomas (endometriotic cysts) which appear as single, multiple, unilateral or bilateral cystic structures. The wall of endometriotic cysts tend to be irregular unlike simple ovarian cysts which have smooth walls. More often than not, the contents of endometriomas show echo patterns compatible with the presence of blood clots, just like in haemorrhagic corpus luteum cysts or ovarian cysts (Figure 7.10). A definitive diagnosis of endometriosis, however, depends on direct visualisation of the lesions at laparoscopy and biopsy could be required in equivocal cases.

### *Ovarian cysts*

Cystic lesions in the ovary merit further evaluation to ascertain whether they are benign or malignant (Figure 7.11). Ultrasound does not exclude malig-

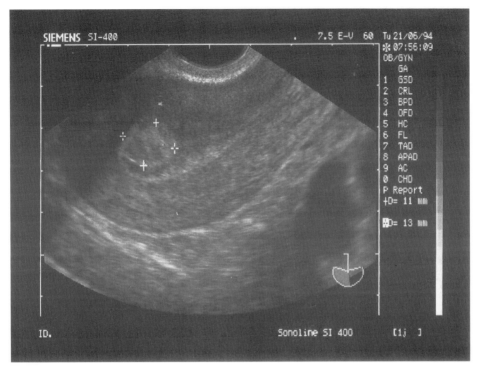

Figure 7.7. Transvaginal sonogram: endometrial polyp in the upper part of the uterine cavity.

nancy completely but may show features which are highly suggestive of a benign nature such as a small size, unilocular and anechoic or hypoechoic appearances of the cyst contents. The ovarian origin of any cyst can be confirmed by demonstrating a rim of ovarian tissue around the cyst. Functional ovarian cysts are commonly found before the menopause and they may be either follicular or luteal (Rajan 1995). Distinguishing features of these cysts include their solitary nature, size rarely in excess of 6 cm and tendency for spontaneous regression (Rajan 1995). Cysts may also arise as result of ovarian stimulation, commonly at the initial (flare-up) phase of gonadotrophin releasing hormone agonist (GnRHa) administration (see Chapter 5). The importance of these benign cysts lies in the fact that they may affect the success of superovulation (Thatcher *et al.* 1989) although this view is by no means unanimous (Karande *et al.* 1990). Rizk *et al.* (1990) analysed the response to superovulation and outcome of *in vitro* fertilisation (IVF) treatment in relation to aspiration or non-aspiration of ovarian cysts that arose before or after initiation of GnRHa therapy. They concluded that aspiration of a unilateral cyst present prior to commencement of GnRHa therapy did not improve follicular

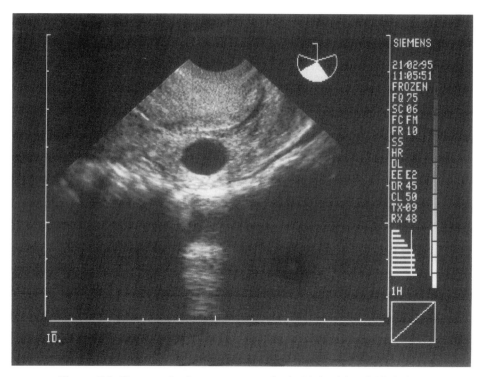

Figure 7.8. Transvaginal sonogram: a single Nabothian follicle in the cervix. The cyst forms when the duct of a cervical gland is blocked by trauma, fibrosis or epithelial overgrowth.

development and recovery of oocytes. When the cyst develops following commencement of agonist use options will include abandonment of the treatment cycle or continuation of the administration of GnRHa until the cyst regresses before commencing gonadotrophin administration. Some would continue with ovarian stimulation while monitoring changes in the size of the cyst.

### *Polycystic ovaries*

Polycystic ovary syndrome (PCOS) classically comprises of infertility, menstrual dysfunction, obesity and hirsutism in the presence of polycystic ovaries (PCO). Experience has however shown that not all these components are present in every female with this syndrome. In fact, PCO may be the only finding in many females. PCOS is rather common and its incidence in the normal population of women has been put at 22% (Polson *et al.* 1988). It is generally believed that this incidence is higher in overweight females than in their normal or underweight counterparts (Amso & Shaw 1992; Duignan 1992;

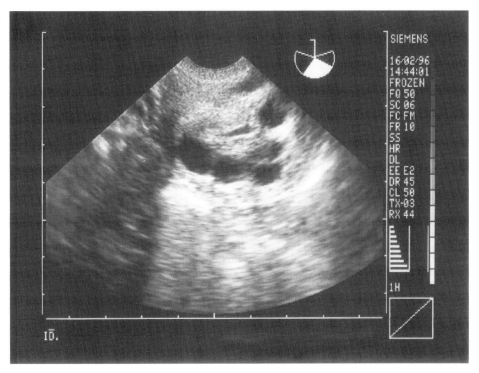

Figure 7.9. Transvaginal sonogram: numerous Nabothian follicles in the cervix which were mistaken for developing ovarian follicles when seen initially during a superovulation cycle.

Hamilton-Fairley et al. 1992). While response in such women to follicular stimulation is largely unpredictable (Amso & Shaw 1992) it is usually excessive (Figure 7.12) with a real risk of the patient developing ovarian hyperstimulation syndrome. This makes it imperative that these females are identified beforehand so that their drug regimen can be manipulated in such a way as to ensure optimal responses without jeopardising their health. Polycystic ovaries tend to be enlarged to a variable extent and have thickened capsules and stroma. A characteristic feature is the presence of numerous follicular cysts which are usually subcapsular in arrangement. Diagnosis of PCOS is by a combination of clinical, ultrasound and endocrinological criteria but ultrasonic features described by Adams et al. (1985) have formed the most important basis for the diagnosis of this condition in many centres in recent years. Diagnosis of PCO is made when at least two of the following three criteria are demonstrated on ultrasound scanning: (1) ovarian volume in excess of 9 cm$^3$, (2) 11 or more follicles measuring 3–8 mm in diameter, and (3) increased stromal density. The typical arrangement of these follicular cysts has been

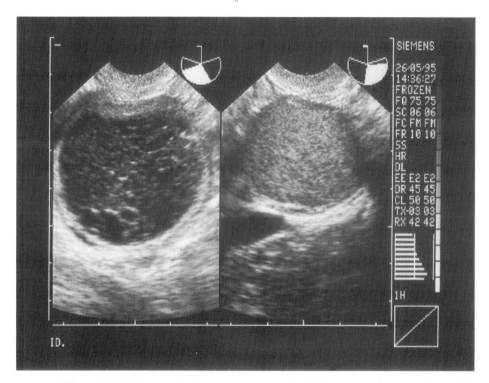

Figure 7.10. Transvaginal sonogram: on the left is an ovarian cyst into which there has been bleeding and on the right is an endometrioma. While the endometrioma presents a homogeneous texture, the haemorrhagic ovarian cyst presents a heterogeneous echo pattern which is mainly cystic with high level internal echoes.

described variously as being in the form of a necklace or a wheel with spokes (Figure 7.13), the spokes formed by compressed ovarian stroma between adjacent follicles. In some cases the follicular cysts are distributed in a random manner throughout the ovary (Figure 7.14).

### *Hydrosalpinges*

It is quite possible to identify the fallopian tubes on ultrasound scanning but this is difficult when the tube is healthy due to its small calibre and tortuous nature unless surrounded by peritoneal fluid. Inflammatory damage to the tubes as a result of infection may occlude the fimbrial end thereby leading to accumulation of tubal secretions within the lumen with a resultant distension of the tube (Figure 7.15). A hydrosalpinx is much easier to detect and typically appears as a fusiform anechoic adnexal mass, tapering towards or enlarging away from the uterus with no detectable peristaltic movements (Fleischer &

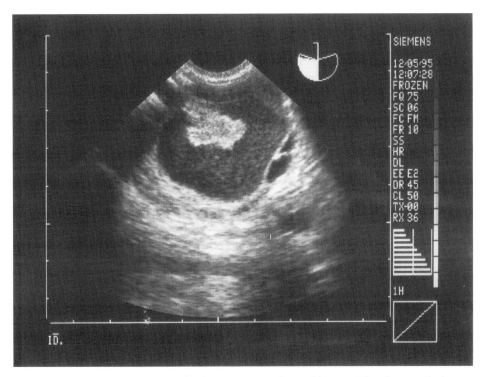

Figure 7.11. Transvaginal sonogram: dermoid cyst. The hyperechoic area represents solid contents of the cyst such as cartilage, hair and teeth.

Entman 1991b). Recent findings indicate that the presence of hydrosalpinges jeopardises the outcome of assisted conception treatment. Although the exact mechanism is not clear at present it is most likely to be related to toxic factors contained in the hydrosalpingeal fluid. Detrimental effects may be exerted during folliculogenesis and/or on the endometrium, the latter situation impairing implantation. A previous history of pelvic inflammatory disease or ectopic pregnancy may alert the clinician and sonographer to the presence of tubal damage. If ultrasound scanning reveals any suspicion of tubal pathology, full evaluation must be carried out to ascertain the suitability of the patient for IUI which requires intact normal tubes for optimal results.

### Hysterosalpingo contrast sonography

Hysterosalpingography (HSG), laparoscopy and chromotubation have been used in a complementary manner for many years in assessing the integrity of the uterine cavity and patency of the fallopian tubes. Many would regard HSG as a primary screening tool while laparoscopic evaluation is needed to confirm

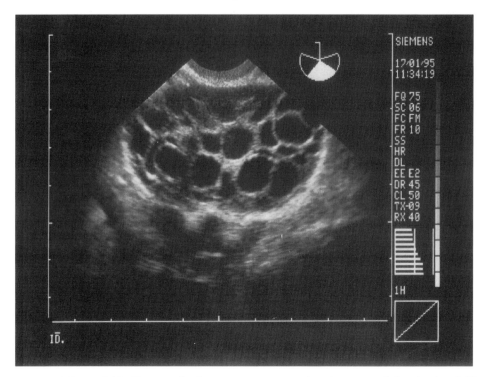

Figure 7.12. Transvaginal sonogram: ovary showing several developing follicles. There has been an exaggerated response to superovulation in a patient with polycystic ovaries.

a preliminary impression of tubal blockage by the lack of spillage of dye from the fimbrial end of the tube. Furthermore, laparoscopy provides useful information regarding the disposition of the pelvic organs and pathology such as endometriosis and adhesions. These investigations have well-known shortcomings. Laparoscopy is invasive, invariably carried out under general anaesthesia and hospitalisation is usually required for at least a few hours. There is always a risk of complications from the surgical procedure and anaesthesia and it is more expensive than HSG. HSG itself exposes the patient to radiation, no matter how small. Some people may exhibit anaphylaxis to the iodinated contrast material that is injected.

It is logical that following the introduction of ultrasonography into infertility management there would be attempts to develop methods for visualising the uterine cavity and verifying patency of the tubes with the ultrasound scanner. Hysterosalpingo contrast sonography (HyCoSy) came into being as a result of early observations that fluid in the uterine cavity and fallopian tubes enhanced the imaging of these structures (Deichert 1994a). Unsatisfactory performance of early contrast media such as normal saline and Ringer's lactate led to the

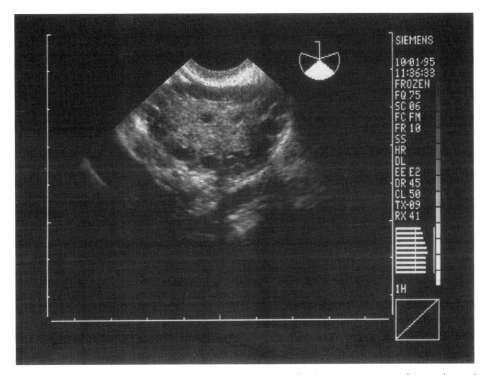

Figure 7.13. Transvaginal sonogram: typical appearances of a polycystic ovary. There is a thick echogenic ovarian stroma with numerous follicular cysts which are arranged around the periphery giving a 'necklace' type appearance.

evaluation of Echovist (Schering Health Care Ltd, West Sussex, UK) which is a suspension of microparticles of galactose in 20% galactose solution. When the mixture is shaken microscopic air bubbles form thereby imparting a strongly echogenic quality to the medium (Deichert 1994a).

HyCoSy is performed with the aid of a purpose made-catheter which is passed into the uterine cavity and retained by inflating the balloon. The uterine cavity is first of all filled by slowly injecting 2–5 ml of Echovist. The injection is continued slowly in increments of not more than 1–2 ml while monitoring the flow of the contrast medium through the fallopian tubes with the transvaginal probe. Tubal patency is diagnosed if continuous flow of this medium in the intramural area, isthmus or ampulla of the fallopian tube is observed for at least 5–10 seconds using B-mode scanning (Deichert 1994a) or there is spillage of the contrast medium from the fimbrial end of the tube. Pulsed wave Doppler studies may be used in cases where two-dimensional imaging is difficult. Tubal patency in such situations is shown by the presence of a typical flow velocity waveform (Deichert 1994a).

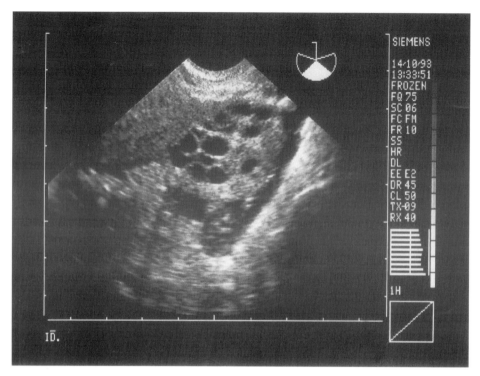

Figure 7.14. Transvaginal sonogram: polycystic ovary with the follicular cysts scattered throughout the substance of the ovary (see Figure 7.13).

HyCoSy is well tolerated (Degenhardt 1994; Deichert 1994b) with adverse effects being recorded in just 4% of patients. Such problems include pain from distension of the uterus and fallopian tubes, vasovagal reactions (sweating, dizziness, nausea and vomiting) and ascending genital tract infection. Echovist should not be used when there is a history of galactosaemia. HyCoSy should be avoided during pregnancy and in pelvic inflammatory disease. Studies so far have shown the sensitivity and specificity of this technique to be quite close to that of HSG and laparoscopy and dye test (Campbell 1994) but further information is needed to determine its exact role in the evaluation of infertility. At present it is tentatively positioned as a primary screening tool similar to HSG but cheaper and free from radiation worries and the potential risk of anaphylaxis. Laparoscopy will still be required for the complete evaluation of an infertile female. The reader is referred to the proceedings of a workshop on this subject (Campbell 1994).

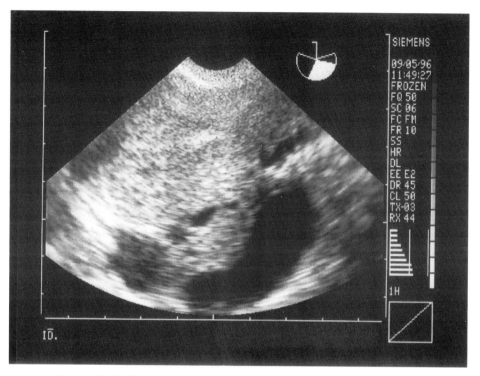

Figure 7.15. Transvaginal sonogram: typical appearances of a hydrosalpinx. The ovary lies between the uterus and the hydrosalpinx.

### Monitoring follicular development

Developing ovarian follicles are first detected by transvaginal ultrasonography when they measure between 2 and 3 mm in diameter, and by abdominal scanning slightly later at 3–5 mm. In the natural cycle usually only one follicle continues to grow while others stop growing and this selection of the dominant follicle takes place before day 5 of the ovarian cycle. Subsequent growth of this dominant follicle is approximately linear (2–3 mm/day) and ovulation occurs after the follicle reaches 18–24 mm in diameter. The use of ovarian stimulants prevents selection of a dominant follicle; rather the hormonal milieu is changed to favour the development of more follicles (Figures 7.16 and 7.17) which subsequently ovulate in response to an endogenous surge of luteinising hormone (LH) or the administration of human chorionic gonadotrophin (hCG) which acts as a surrogate LH surge. Growth of follicles following ovarian stimulation depends on the type of stimulant used and the dose but this is significantly modified by other factors such as the age and build of the patient, and pre-existing conditions such as polycystic ovaries. During transvaginal scanning, it should always be borne in mind that other structures may

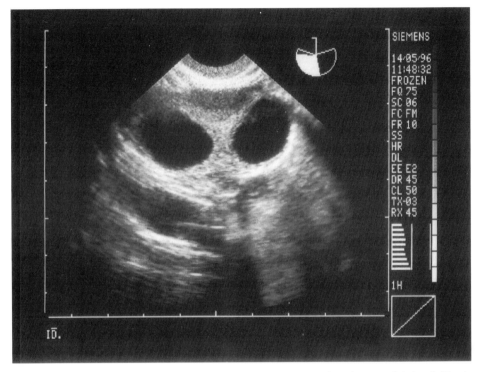

Figure 7.16. Transvaginal sonogram: ovary showing multiple follicular development in response to superovulation induction. This is preparatory to intrauterine insemination and the aim is for production of three and certainly not more than five mature fertilisable oocytes (see Chapter 6).

at times be mistaken for ovarian follicles such as cross-sections of pelvic blood vessels (Figure 7.18), bowel loops (Figure 7.19), hydrosalpinx and ovarian cysts. Rotating the angle of the transducer will often show the longitudinal sections of vessels. Furthermore, arterial pulsation will be seen on the scan. When observed long enough, peristaltic movements are usually seen in bowel loops and the bowel contents are echogenic. Diagnostic features of hydrosalpinges and ovarian cysts have already been described in preceding sections. The growing follicle is not usually uniformly spherical, especially when many are developing at the same time, so the internal diameter is measured in three planes and the mean value computed.

The ability to monitor follicular growth and predict precisely the time of ovulation is pivotal to the running of a successful assisted conception programme because it allows artificial insemination or oocyte recovery at optimal time periods. Methods utilised in monitoring follicular development are based on the results of studies seeking direct and indirect measures of ovarian activity in the natural cycle or following ovarian stimulation. It has been established

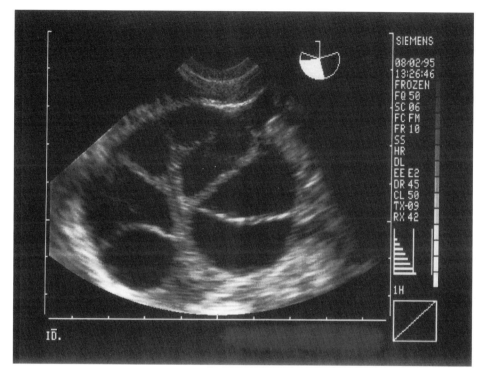

Figure 7.17. Transvaginal sonogram: ovary showing development of several follicles during an in vitro fertilisation treatment cycle. Superovulation here aims at production of an average of ten oocytes. The oocytes are aspirated from the follicles just prior to ovulation.

that plasma oestrogen concentration correlates closely with the stage of development of the dominant follicle in a normal unstimulated ovarian cycle; as the follicular size increases, so also does the amount of oestrogen it produces (Hackeloer et al. 1979). This correlation is however lower in stimulated cycles as the plasma oestrogen concentration in such cases reflects the total output of all developing follicles irrespective of their size. For example, a patient with several small sized follicles may have the same plasma oestrogen concentration as another who has fewer but larger follicles. Ultrasound scanning, in contrast, provides a more direct assessment of follicular development. Both number and size of follicles can be determined and their growth rate followed more accurately, thereby helping to determine the optimum time to trigger ovulation, especially in cycles conducted after pituitary downregulation. Another problem with endocrinological monitoring of superovulation is the disruption of patients' social and work routines because they have to report to the unit at close intervals for blood samples to be withdrawn, usually in the morning, and come back later or ring for the results before having further gonadotrophin

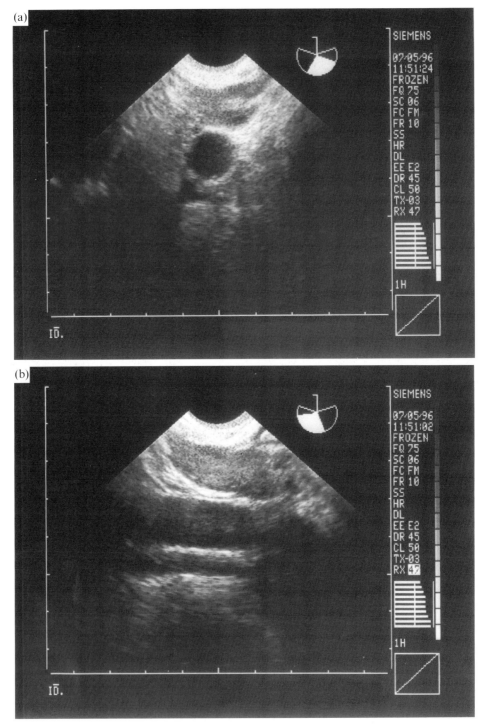

Figure 7.18. Transvaginal sonogram. (a) Transverse section of a pelvic blood vessel which may be confused with an ovarian follicle; (b) however, rotation of the transducer reveals this to be a blood vessel. The artery, which runs beneath this vein, is seen to pulsate and is of smaller calibre than the vein.

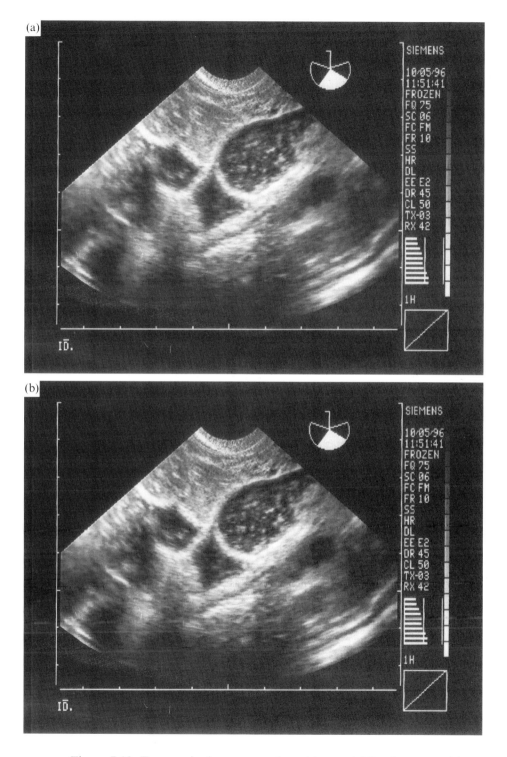

Figure 7.19. Transvaginal sonogram: bowel loops. (a) In close apposition to the uterus. Echogenic bowel contents are more clearly seen in (b). Peristaltic waves are usually noted at intervals

injections. For many years a combination of oestradiol assay and ultrasound monitoring of follicular development was used in an attempt to improve the timing of ovulation, however, recent trends have marked a move away from the use endocrinological monitoring methods. Instead sole use is now made of ultrasound scanning especially in cycles employing GnRHa to suppress the endogenous surge of LH. Reports from centres using this monitoring strategy have shown that this is still compatible with normal pregnancy rates with the incidence of ovarian hyperstimulation syndrome still being within the normal range (Wikland 1992; Golan *et al.* 1994; Tsirigotis *et al.* 1995). Accounts on the use of ultrasound and luteinising hormone detection kits to monitor ovarian response to superovulation in IUI cycles are presented in Chapter 6.

### Diagnosis of ovulation

Ultrasonographic diagnosis of ovulation is easiest when made in relation to a cycle that has been monitored prospectively. This is because the prior existence of follicular development has to be documented as well as optimal growth patterns and the achievement of a certain range of pre-ovulatory follicular dimension. Workers who have closely monitored peri-ovulatory events have demonstrated the cumulus oophorus in the 24 hours preceding ovulation in up to 65% of follicles (Hackeloer *et al.* 1979). Ovulation itself is commonly observed as a sudden escape of fluid from the mature follicle, an event of which is followed, within an hour, by bleeding into the follicle and the formation of the corpus haemorrhagicum (Blumenfeld *et al.* 1990). In the routine clinical situation, these events are rarely observed as patients are scanned for just a few minutes every day or two. The most commonly sought features in such circumstances are the presence of fluid in the pouch of Douglas, echogenic areas within follicle(s) previously known to be echo free, and ill-defined outline of the follicle(s) (Blumenfeld *et al.* 1990). It is important to document ovulation whenever possible in an IUI treatment cycle in order to help shed more light on the optimal timing of insemination, and the longevity of inseminated spermatozoa and ovulated oocytes. Usually, features of ovulation are sought for at the time of the first and second inseminations.

### Sonographic evaluation of cyclical endometrial activity

In the normal course of events the mammalian endometrium goes through a regular cycle of proliferative and secretory changes followed by degeneration, sloughing off and/or regression. The primate corpus luteum has a lifespan of between 14 and 16 days with a state of functional regression being entered by days 23–24 of the cycle (Bonney & Franks 1990). Fertilisation of the oocyte, which is released at the end of the proliferative phase, results in an interruption of this cycle. Degeneration of the endometrium is prevented; rather, further growth and development occurs thereby providing a favourable environment for the implantation and nurture of the embryo. The best known agent responsible for this change is chorionic gonadotrophin which is secreted by the embryo and stimulates the corpus luteum to increase its production of ovarian steroids. Other embryonic pre-implantation signals have now been identified. Maintenance of the endometrium is an important component of maternal recognition of pregnancy, which as defined by Lenton & Woodward (1988) is 'the specific biochemical changes in the maternal organism that only occur as a consequence of the presence of an early pregnancy'. Such recognition is needed to prevent menstruation, prepare the endometrium for implantation, assist the process of implantation, prevent rejection of the embryo, nourish the embryo, prevent excessive invasion of maternal tissue by the trophoblast, allow pregnancy to proceed and to stimulate changes in the maternal physiology that will result in optimal growth and survival of the conceptus. A requirement for optimal recognition and support of pregnancy is an adequate prior degree of exposure to oestrogens and progesterone in the proliferative and luteal phases of the normal menstrual cycle. Without this, endometrial receptivity will be insufficient leading to failed implantation and early spontaneous abortion (Bonney & Franks 1990). Another consideration is that of synchronisation of developmental changes in the embryo with maturation of the endometrium. Successful implantation will only occur within a narrow time range in most mammals and the term 'implantation window' has been used for this period of receptivity. Much still remains to be learnt about this important aspect of reproductive physiology which also has a strong bearing on the assisted reproductive technologies.

There have been attempts to ascertain whether there are peculiar endometrial sonographic features that can be used to predict the occurrence of pregnancy in natural or stimulated cycles. This search has come about because of the well-known fact that implantation will usually only take place if the endometrium has reached a certain stage of development. The expectation is that endometrial development will have ultrasonographic correlates which can be easily recognised and hopefully quantified for the purpose of documentation, research and comparison of findings from different centres. In so doing the most favourable configuration would be determined and applied clinically to improve implantation and pregnancy rates. This prospective assessment method is appealing because it is non-invasive and does not cause any deleterious effects on the endometrium, unlike biopsy for example, which causes bleeding, tissue damage and inflammatory responses that jeopardise nidation in the index menstrual or assisted conception treatment cycle. Furthermore, it offers the prospect of manipulating the treatment protocol in tandem with sequential ultrasonic findings in order to achieve the optimal outcome in that same cycle.

The two most common features that are presently assessed are endometrial thickness and reflectivity (also called texture or quality). From a very thin layer measuring about 3 mm during menstrual bleeding (Fried 1995), the endometrium gradually increases in thickness during the follicular phase and measures between 10 and 14 mm at the time of ovulation (Forrest et al. 1988; Blumenfeld 1990) with further increases occurring in the luteal phase. Endometrial growth in the follicular phase is mainly due to proliferation of cellular elements while in the luteal phase secretory activities predominate with the production, storage and secretion of mucin by the endometrial glands. There is also deposition of glycogen in the endometrium in addition to congestion and oedema. Endometrial texture or reflectivity also changes during the menstrual cycle. Various descriptive terms have been applied to these changes and there is as yet no agreement on terminology. The sonographic image of the endometrium has a multilayer appearance (triple line) in the late follicular phase while in the luteal phase echogenicity of the endometrium increases until it becomes uniformly hyperechogenic by the mid-luteal phase (Alam & Hess 1993). The triple line pattern is composed of hyperechogenic lines that mark the junction between the endometrium and the myometrium on each side, the hypoechogenic endometrial tissue lying between these lines, and the central line that demarcates the apposed endometrial surfaces of the uterus. The sonographic endometrial pattern of the follicular phase can be further subdivided into various grades which together form a continuum of changes occurring from the beginning of the follicular phase until the peri-ovulatory period (Figures 7.20–7.24). It is regarded as an unfavourable sign if an earlier sonographic grade persists into the late follicular phase. The criteria we have adopted for grading endometrial quality (texture, reflectivity) at the London Gynaecology and Fertility Centre are as follows:

> Grade C: an entirely homogenous hyperechoic endometrium. This may be noted in the first few days of the menstrual period before the endometrium is shed completely.
>
> Grade B: a multilayer endometrial pattern with the bulk of the endometrium exhibiting an echogenicity that is similar to or less than that of the myometrium.
>
> Grade A: a multilayer endometrial pattern with the bulk of the endometrium exhibiting an echogenicity that is slightly more than that of the myometrium. This is the most desirable endometrial grading to have at the time of ovulation.

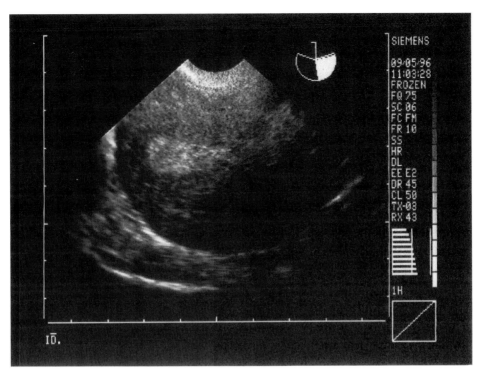

Figure 7.20. Transvaginal sonogram: Grade C endometrial texture found at commencement of a menstrual period. This is actually the feature seen during the luteal phase of the menstrual cycle.

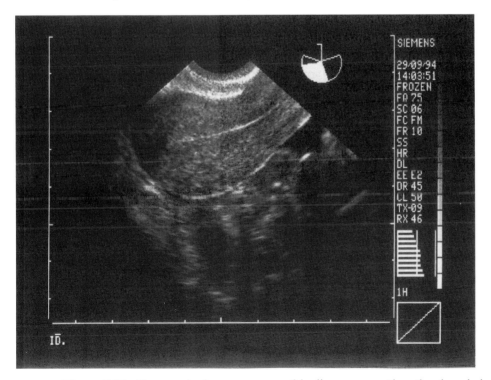

Figure 7.21. Transvaginal sonogram: a thin line representing the denuded endometrium at the end of menstrual bleeding.

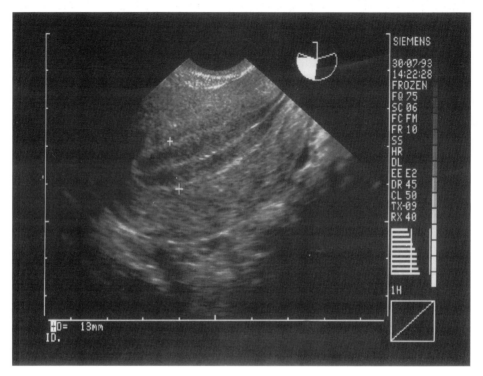

Figure 7.22. Transvaginal sonogram: Grade B endometrium. A triple-line pattern is seen within which the endometrium demonstrates an echogenicity that is less than that of the myometrium. The endometrial thickness at this time is 13 mm.

Conflicting results have been reported by various workers who have evaluated the ability of these endometrial parameters to predict conception in natural or stimulated cycles. Accounts of these reports and suitable references can be found in Blumenfeld et al. (1990), Tan et al. (1992), Wikland (1992) and Alam & Hess (1993). The general impression, however, seems to be that the chances of conception improve with an increase in endometrial thickness and a preovulatory endometrium of more than 10 mm in thickness; Grade A quality is the most favourable feature. It is quite obvious that there are many confounding factors which have to be identified and corrected for before data on the correlation of endometrial appearances with conception rates can be interpreted with confidence. Endometrial receptivity is not the only factor that influences nidation and the establishment of pregnancy. Several other factors, including those that influence embryo viability, have significant effects too. Finally, reports on endometrial response to circulating ovarian steroid levels in unstimulated as well as stimulated cycles suggest that there is a maximal response by the endometrium which is achieved in the natural cycle and is not

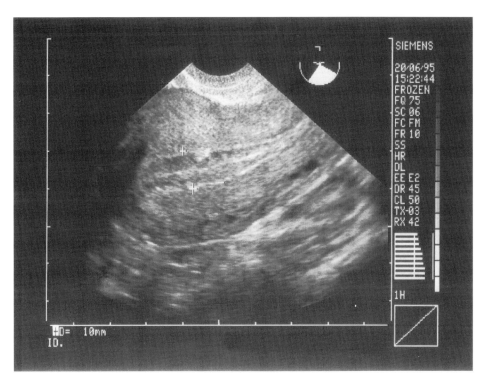

Figure 7.23. Transvaginal sonogram: endometrium showing what can be classified as B/A texture, i.e. midway between Grades A and B. The endometrial thickness in this case is 10 mm.

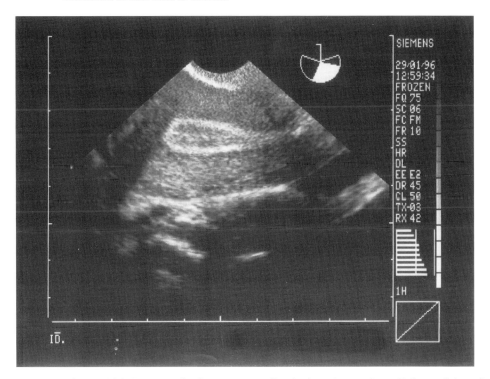

Figure 7.24. Transvaginal sonogram: Grade A endometrium. Echogenicity of the endometrium is slightly more than that of the surrounding myometrium.

increased further by the high steroid levels found in stimulated cycles (Tan *et al.* 1992).

### Conclusion

Pelvic ultrasonography plays a crucial role in the management of infertile couples. It assists in the diagnosis of pelvic pathology as well as systemic disease with pelvic markers such as PCOS. Assisted conception treatment is conducted more efficiently and safely when ultrasonography is utilised as a monitoring tool. The information provided in this chapter has a direct bearing on the use of IUI in the management of infertility in couples. Ultrasonography has other applications in infertility management which have not been presented here. Recovery of oocytes for IVF for example, is carried out almost exclusively nowadays with ultrasound-directed ovarian puncture. Transfer of embryos into the uterine cavity as well the fallopian tubes is performed by some practitioners under ultrasonic guidance. Although deposition of the inseminated sperm suspension into the uterine cavity can be confirmed ultrasonographically (Blumenfeld *et al.* 1990) it is not clear how useful this is in practice as it can be safely inferred that uterine insemination has taken place when there is complete expulsion of the fluid from the syringe and catheter without significant back flow or pericervical leakage occurring. Colour Doppler ultrasonography has been applied to the study of uterine and ovarian arterial blood flow in infertile women and those having assisted conception treatment (Tan *et al.* 1992; Wikland 1992) but the role of this investigative tool has not been fully evaluated at present. Similarly, studies of endometrial peristalsis are still in their infancy (Allabadiah 1995). Following conception ultrasound scanning provides useful information on zygosity and can be applied to the diagnosis of problems such as ectopic pregnancy, higher order multiple pregnancy and abortion (Figures 7.25–7.27).

### Acknowledgement

We thank Mrs Nahid Amiri, DMU, for her invaluable assistance during the preparation of this chapter.

### References

Abramovici H., Faktor J. H. & Pascal B. (1983) Congenital uterine malformations as indication for cervical suture (cerclage) in habitual abortion and premature delivery. *International Journal of Fertility* **28**, 161–164.

Adams J., Polson D. W., Abdulwahid N., Morris D. V., Franks S., Mason H. D., Tucker M., Price J. & Jacobs H. S. (1985) Multifollicular ovaries: clinical and

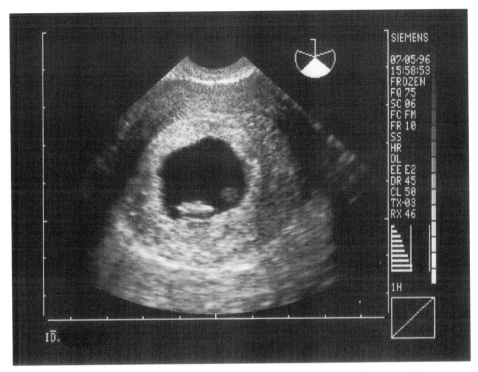

Figure 7.25. Transvaginal sonogram: singleton intrauterine gestation.

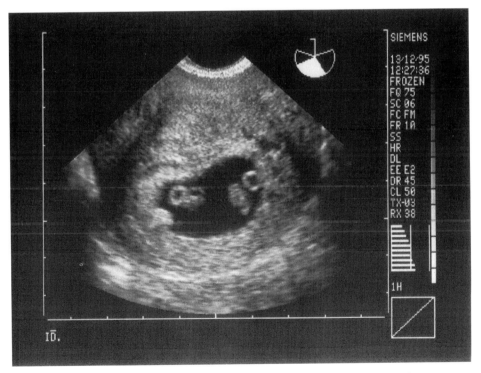

Figure 7.26. Transvaginal sonogram: monochorionic twin gestation.

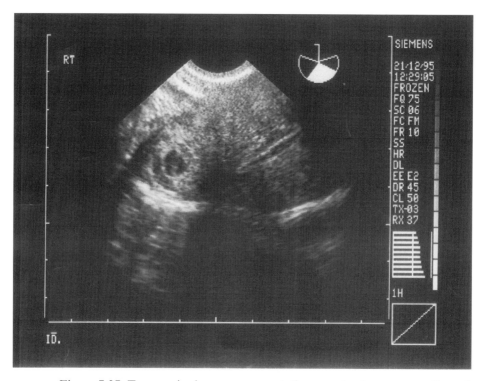

Figure 7.27. Transvaginal sonogram: gestation sac clearly seen away from the endometrial cavity; a cornual ectopic pregnancy.

endocrine features and response to pulsatile gonadotrophin releasing hormone. *Lancet* **2**, 1375–1378.

Alam V. A. & Hess R. B. (1993) Echographic visualization of the endometrium: a marker for fertility? In: *Annual Progress in Reproductive Medicine: 1993.* (R. H. Asch, J. W. W. Studd, eds), Parthenon Publishing Group, Canforth, pp. 59–64.

Allabadiah G. (1995) Transvaginal sonography in the study of endometrial physiology and pathology. In: *Infertility and Transvaginal Sonography; Current Concepts.* (S. Desai, G. Allahbadia, eds), Jaypee Brothers Medical Publishers Ltd, New Delhi, pp. 212–218.

Amso N. N. & Shaw R. W. (1992) New frontiers in assisted reproduction. In: *Gynaecology.* (R. Shaw, P. Soutter, S. Stanton, eds), first edition, Churchill Livingstone, Edinburgh, pp. 231–248.

Ansbacher R. (1983) Uterine anomalies and future pregnancies. *Clinics in Perinatology* **10**, 295–304.

Bonney R. C. & Franks S. (1990) The endocrinology of implantation and early pregnancy. *Baillière's Clinical Endocrinology and Metabolism* **4**, 207–231.

Blumenfeld Z., Yoffe N. & Bronshtein M. (1990) Transvaginal sonography in infertility and assisted reproduction. *Obstetrical and Gynecological Survey* **46**, 36–48.

Campbell S. (1994) The future of HyCoSy in infertility investigation. In: *Viewpoints in Medicine: Infertility Investigation in Europe and the Future Role of Hysterosalpingo Contrast Sonography (HyCoSy).* (S. Campbell, chairman), Cambridge Medical Publications, Worthing, pp. 34–36.

Degenhardt F. (1994) Clinical results with HyCoSy: Study 2. In: *Viewpoints in Medicine: Infertility Investigation in Europe and the Future Role of Hysterosalpingo Contrast Sonography (HyCoSy)*. (S. Campbell, chairman), Cambridge Medical Publications, Worthing, pp. 24–25.

Deichart U. (1994a) Hysterosalpingo contrast sonography (HyCoSy): a new technique for assessing tubal patency. In: *Viewpoints in Medicine: Infertility Investigation in Europe and the Future Role of Hysterosalpingo Contrast Sonography (HyCoSy)*. (S. Campbell, chairman), Cambridge Medical Publications, Worthing, pp. 19–22.

Deichart U. (1994b) Clinical results with HyCoSy: Study 3. In: *Viewpoints in Medicine: Infertility Investigation in Europe and the Future Role of Hysterosalpingo Contrast Sonography (HyCoSy)*. (S. Campbell, chairman), Cambridge Medical Publications, Worthing, pp. 25–27.

Duignan N. M. (1992) Hirsutism and virilization. In: *Gynaecology*. (R. Shaw, P. Soutter, S. Stanton, eds), first edition, Churchill Livingstone, Edinburgh, pp. 313–324.

Fleischer A. C. & Entman S. S. (1991a) Sonographic evaluation of the uterus and related disorders. In: *The Principles and Practice of Ultrasonography in Obstetrics and Gynecology*. (A. C. Fleischer, R. Romero, F. A. Manning, P. Jeanty, A. E. James Jr, eds), fourth edition, Appleton and Lange, Norwalk, pp. 565–595.

Fleischer A. C. & Entman S. S. (1991b) Sonographic evaluation of pelvic masses with transabdominal and transvaginal scanning. In: *The Principles and Practice of Ultrasonography in Obstetrics and Gynecology*. (A. C. Fleischer, R. Romero, F. A. Manning, P. Jeanty, A. E. James Jr, eds), fourth edition, Appleton and Lange, Norwalk, pp. 537–556.

Forrest T. S., Elyaderm M. K., Muilenburg M. I., Bewtrac C., Kable W. T. & Sullivan P. (1988) Cyclical endometrial changes: ultrasonic assessment with histologic correlation. *Radiology* **167**, 233–237.

Fried A. M. (1995) Transvaginal sonography of the uterus. In: *Infertility and Transvaginal Sonography; Current Concepts*. (S. Desai, G. Allahbadia, eds), Jaypee Brothers Medical Publishers Ltd, New Delhi, pp. 208–211.

Golan A., Herman A., Soffer Y., Bukovsky I. & Ron-El R. (1994) Ultrasonic control without hormone determination for ovulation induction in in vitro fertilization/embryo transfer with gonadotrophin-releasing hormone analogue and human menopausal gonadotrophin. *Human Reproduction* **9**, 1631–1633.

Golan A., Langer R., Bukovsky I. & Caspi E. (1989) Congenital anomalies of the mullerian system. *Fertility and Sterility* **51**, 747–755.

Hackeloer B. J. (1977) The ultrasonic demonstration of follicular development during the normal menstrual cycle and after hormone stimulation. In: *Recent Advances in Ultrasound Diagnosis*. (A. Kurjak, ed.), Excerpta Medica, Amsterdam, pp. 122–128.

Hackeloer B. J., Fleming R., Robinson H. P., Adam A. H. & Coutts J. R. T. (1979) Correlation of ultrasonic and endocrinologic assessment of human follicular development. *American Journal of Obstetrics and Gynecology* **135**, 122–128.

Hamilton-Fairley D., Kiddy D., Watson H., Paterson C. & Franks S. (1992) Association of moderate obesity with a poor pregnancy outcome in women with polycystic ovary syndrome treated with low dose gonadotrophin. *British Journal of Obstetrics and Gynaecology* **99**, 128–131.

Healy D. L., Lawson S. R., Abbott M., Baird D. T. & Fraser H. M (1986) Towards removing uterine fibroids without surgery: subcutaneous infusion of a luteinizing hormone-releasing hormone agonist commencing in the luteal phase. *Journal of Clinical Endocrinology and Metabolism* **63**, 619–625.

Karande V. C., Scott R. T., Jones G. S. & Muasher S. J. (1990) Non-functional ovarian cysts do not affect ipsilateral or contralateral ovarian performance during in vitro fertilization. *Human Reproduction* **5**, 431–433.

Kratochowil A., Urban G. & Friedrich F. (1972) Ultrasonic tomography of the ovaries. *American Chirugical Gynecology of the Female* **61**, 211–217.

Lenton E. A. & Woodward A. J. (1988) The endocrinology of conception cycles and implantation in women. *Journal of Reproduction and Fertility* (supplement) **36**, 1–15.

Polson D. W., Adams J., Wadsworth J. & Franks S. (1988) Polycystic ovaries – a common finding in normal women. *Lancet* **1**, 870–872.

Rajan R. (1995) Management of ovarian enlargement. In: *Infertility and Transvaginal Sonography; Current Concepts*. (S. Desai, G. Allahbadia, eds), Jaypee Brothers Medical Publishers Ltd, New Delhi, pp. 262–266.

Rizk B., Tan S. L., Kinsgland C., Steer C., Mason B. A. & Campbell S. (1990) Ovarian cyst aspiration and the outcome of in vitro fertilization. *Fertility and Sterility* **54**, 661–664.

Sanfillippo J. S., Wain N. G., Schikler K. N. & Yussman M. A. (1986) Endometriosis in association with uterine anomaly. *American Journal of Obstetrics and Gynecology* **154**, 39–43.

Sanfillippo J. S., Yussman M. A. & Smith O. (1978) Hysterosalpingography in the evaluation of infertility. *Fertility and Sterility* **30**, 636–639.

Tan S. L., Steer C. & Campbell S. (1992) Ultrasound in the monitoring of assisted conception. In: *A Textbook of In Vitro Fertilization and Assisted Reproduction*. (P. R. Brinsden, P. A. Rainsbury, eds), The Parthenon Publishing Group, Carnforth, pp. 127–138.

Thatcher S. S., Jones E. & DeCherney A. H. (1989) Ovarian cysts decrease the success of controlled ovarian stimulation and in vitro fertilization. *Fertility and Sterility* **52**, 812–816.

Tindall V. R. (1987) Malformations and maldevelopments of the genital tract. In *Jeffcoate's Principles of Gynaecology*, fifth edition, Butterworth & Co. (Publishers) Ltd, London, pp. 138–158.

Tsirigotis M., Hutchon S., Yazdani N. & Craft I. (1995) The value of oestradiol estimations in controlled ovarian hyperstimulation cycles. *Human Reproduction* **10**, 972–973 (letter).

Wikland M. (1992) Vaginal ultrasound in assisted reproduction. *Baillières Clinical Obstetrics and Gynaecology* **6**, 283–296.

# 8
# Semen analysis and sperm preparation

STEVEN D. FLEMING, GODWIN I. MENIRU, JENNY A. HALL and SIMON B. FISHEL

### Introduction

A detailed semen analysis is required as part of the initial diagnostic work-up of the infertile couple before the decision for intrauterine insemination (IUI) or any other management option is made. Following acceptance into the programme, semen is next produced about 2 hours before the proposed time of insemination so as to allow enough time for its preparation. Several methods have been described for preparing semen to be used for assisted conception treatments. The decision on which particular method to use often depends on the experience of the workers but the quality of the semen sample is also a major determinant. Methods for preparing very poor semen samples will not be described here as we believe that such patients should be treated with in vitro fertilisation or any of its variants rather than with IUI.

### Production of specimen

Semen is produced by masturbation following 3–5 days of ejaculatory abstinence. Sterile, wide-mouth, non-toxic plastic containers are used and they should be labelled with patient identifying information. The whole of an ejaculate may be collected in a single container or split between two receptacles. The latter method of collection aims at separating the spermatozoa-rich initial portion of the ejaculate from the latter part that tends to contain more seminal fluid (MacLeod & Hotchkiss 1942; Farris & Murphy 1960; Perez-Pelaez & Cohen 1965) thereby increasing the efficacy of sperm preparation methods. Furthermore, it prevents spermatozoa coming into contact with a large amount of seminal fluid which at times may have anti-fertility components.

The male partner of the infertile couple is instructed in clear terms on how to produce a split ejaculate; he is told to direct the first one or two spurts of ejaculate into a pot marked '1' and the rest into pot '2'. Collection of semen is usually with multipurpose plastic containers in most units and split ejaculates are produced into two specimen pots which are held together with an adhesive tape. Application of the tape is an awkward process and when bound in such a manner it is difficult unscrewing the caps which lie very close together and impede each others movement. The numbers '1' and '2' are written on the caps of these containers with marking pens to aid correct replacement on the respective container but patients still mix them up quite often. A new range of containers suitable for collection of whole and spilt ejaculates have now been designed (world-wide patent pending status) (G.I. Meniru & M.O. Meniru; unpublished results). Finally, on-site production of the specimen is preferable as this ensures that fresh samples arrive at the laboratory within a short time of ejaculation.

Visual aids such as erotic magazines or video recordings should be placed in the room for those who require them. If the man finds it impossible to masturbate within the hospital premises he is asked to do so at home and bring in the specimen within an hour of production, avoiding exposure of the sample to extreme weather conditions. The pots are preferably transported to hospital in an inner coat pocket.

In extreme cases where he is unable to produce semen on demand, even in familiar home surroundings, cryopreservation of samples produced at will before and/or during his wife's follicular stimulation, is carried out. The required number of ampoules (or straws) of cryopreserved semen can then be thawed and prepared when she is ready for insemination. Great tact and compassion are both needed when dealing with these men. Enough time should be spent explaining the requirements and reasons for making them. Each couple should be informed in advance of the need to produce semen on site, but wishes regarding an alternative location for masturbation should be acceded to while making sure the dialogue is properly documented. It has to be realised that some men may find it off-putting, being asked to masturbate on demand in a clinical and unfamiliar environment.

### Semen analysis

Despite well-known limitations, semen analysis is still the main laboratory technique used in obtaining indirect indices of a man's fertility potential. Standardisation of techniques is of key importance as it enables meaningful comparison of results from different centres. The World Health Organization has championed this approach for many years and the latest manual (WHO 1992) should be available in every unit where semen analysis is performed.

Table 8.1. *Normal values of standard semen analysis*

| | |
|---|---|
| Liquefaction | Complete within 60 minutes at room temperature |
| Appearance | Homogeneous, grey opalescent |
| Odour | 'Fresh' and characteristic |
| Consistency | Leaves pipette as discrete droplets |
| Volume | 2 ml or more |
| pH | 7.2–8.0 |
| Sperm concentration | $20 \times 10^6$ spermatozoa/ml or more |
| Total sperm count | $40 \times 10^6$ spermatozoa per ejaculate or more |
| Motility | 50% or more with forward progression (categories 'a' and 'b') or 25% or more with rapid progression (category 'a') within 60 minutes of ejaculation |
| Morphology | 30% or more with normal forms |
| Vitality | 75% or more live |
| White blood cells | Fewer than $1 \times 10^6$/ml |
| Immunobead test | Fewer than 20% spermatozoa with adherent particles |
| MAR test | Fewer than 10% spermatozoa with adherent particles |

*Source:* World Health Organization (1992).

Additional tests are left to the discretion of scientific and clinical staff with the proviso that these tests should be audited on a continuous basis in order to confirm their usefulness in the unit. Results of sperm morphology assessment in which strict criteria are used in determining normality or otherwise have been shown to correlate very closely with the outcome of some assisted conception treatments (Oehninger & Kruger 1995) but not others such as intracytoplasmic sperm injection (Hall *et al.* 1993; Fleming *et al.* 1994). An outline of the technique of semen analysis will be described here. More details will be found in the WHO (1992) manual. Currently acceptable normal values are shown in Table 8.1. We recommend use of the Makler sperm counting chamber (Figure 8.1) as it gives a consistent depth of fluid under the coverslip and in so doing reduces the intra- and interobserver variability that plagues most other counting chambers. Results obtained from analysis of the two portions of the split ejaculate are added and divided by two in order to get the result for the whole ejaculate.

### Steps in semen analysis

1. On receiving the semen sample, confirm that the patient's name corresponds to that written on the specimen container label and the laboratory request form.
2. Note the time of production and determine whether the semen has liquefied

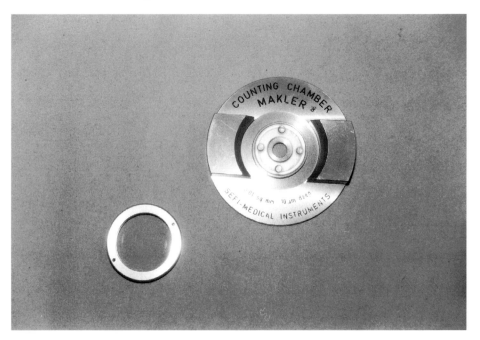

Figure 8.1. The Makler sperm counting chamber reduces both intra- and interobserver variability in the results of sperm concentration determination.

completely or not. If liquefaction has occurred, proceed with the analysis. If not, let the container of semen rest on the bench at room temperature for complete liquefaction of the sample to occur. If this does not happen within 30 minutes place the sample in the incubator for another 30 minutes. If at the end of this time it is still viscous, aspirate and expel the semen repeatedly through a 19 (French) gauge hypodermic needle using a syringe. The syringe should not have any rubber components. An alternative is to place the container on its side upon an automated roller, ensuring the cap is tightly sealed.

3. Observe the appearance of the sample and note any abnormal odour emanating from it.
4. Measure the volume of the ejaculate with a sterile graduated pipette and check for its consistency by letting it drop slowly from the pipette. The pH should also be measured by smearing a drop of semen on pH paper and observing the colour change and its equivalent pH reading.
5. Gently swirl the semen around in the container to ensure it is properly mixed before withdrawing 5 µl of the sample with a micropipettor and placing it on a plain glass slide. Carefully place a coverslip on top of this drop and apply gentle pressure with the thumb so as to spread it well and obtain a thin layer of semen. Any excess fluid escaping from the edges of the coverslip should be dabbed away with clean tissue paper. The slide is examined under the micro-

*Semen analysis and sperm preparation* 133

scope with the motility and progression of 100 spermatozoa being estimated using the WHO (1992) guide:
- a rapid progressive motility
- b slow or sluggish motility
- c non-progressive motility
- d immotility

6. Check for the presence of agglutination (sticking to one another) of motile spermatozoa.
7. Examine the morphology of 100 spermatozoa using the Tygerberg strict criteria (Kruger *et al.* 1987; Menkveld *et al.* 1990) after staining with the Diff Quik staining kit (Baxter Dade Diagnostics AG, Dubingen, Switzerland) as follows:

### *Staining technique (Fleming et al. 1994)*

(a) Carefully wash the slides to be used with 70% (v/v) ethanol and allow to dry.
(b) Place 5 μl of semen onto a prepared slide to create a thin smear.
(c) Air-dry the slide for 3 minutes.
(d) Fix the smear in Diff Quik fixative for 15 seconds.
(e) Stain the smear with Diff Quik solution I for 5 seconds.
(f) Stain the smear with Diff Quik solution II for 5 seconds.
(g) Air-dry the slide in an upright position for about 30 minutes.
(h) Transfer the slides to a fume cupboard and apply coverslips using Xam neutral medium (BDH Laboratory Supplies, Poole, UK).

### *Method of assessment*

(a) Place the slide under a compound light microscope.
(b) Put a drop of oil onto the coverslip and focus through the droplet using the x 100 objective.
(c) Count 100 spermatozoa, grading them according to Figure 8.2 as follows:
   (i) Normal
   (ii) Head piece abnormalities
   (iii) Mid-piece abnormalities
   (iv) Tail-piece abnormalities
   (v) Immature
   (vi) Cytoplasmic droplets

Express the numbers of spermatozoa with each type of abnormality as a percentage of the total count.

8. Determine the concentration of spermatozoa using the Makler counting chamber. Follow carefully the instructions that come with the chamber. Also estimate the concentration of round cells (epithelial cells lining the urethra, immature spermatogenic cells and white blood cells) in the semen sample.

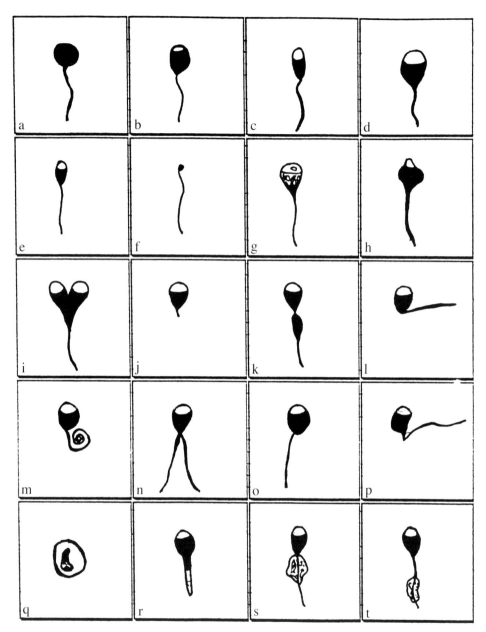

Figure 8.2. Sperm malformations; a: round head/ no acrosome; b: small acrosome; c: elongated head; d: megalo head; e: small head; f: pinhead; g: vacuolated head; h: amorphous head; i: bicephalic; j: loose head; k: amorphous neck; l: broken neck; m: coiled tail; n: double tail; o: abaxial tail attachment; p: multiple defects; q: immature germ cell; r: elongated spermatid; s: proximal cytoplasmic droplet; t: distal cytoplasmic droplet.

Table 8.2. *Sperm preparation methods*

Wash and spin
Wash and swim-up
Swim-up from neat semen (layering)
Self-migration sedimentation
Glass wool column filtration
Glass bead separation
Swim-down through albumin columns
Percoll, PureSperm or ISolate gradient
Nycondenz gradient
Sperm 'entrapment' with Ficoll
Sedimentation under paraffin
Mini-Percoll gradient
Transmembrane migration
Migration across nickel meshes
Sephadex columns

9. The mixed antiglobulin reaction (MAR) test, the immunobead test and optional tests to be performed are as described in the WHO manual (1992) and relevant texts.

**Sperm preparation**

Methods utilised in sperm preparation (Table 8.2) (Mortimer 1994) should be capable of selecting and concentrating the subpopulation of normal motile spermatozoa in the ejaculate. Such methods aim to remove seminal plasma, dead, damaged and abnormal spermatozoa, immature germ cells, bacteria, other cells such as white blood cells, and cellular debris. In so doing, they closely mimic the action of the cervix and cervical mucus on ejaculated semen. Removal of seminal plasma is important because it contains prostaglandins which if inseminated directly into the uterine cavity may stimulate very strong and painful uterine contractions. Furthermore, some other constituents of seminal plasma stabilise the sperm membrane and prevent capacitation (Van der Ven *et al.* 1982) and hyperactivation which normally precede the acrosomal reaction that is necessary for successful sperm invasion of oocyte investments and subsequent fertilisation.

Sterile precautions are observed during sperm preparation for IUI and other assisted conception treatments. Thorough hand washing, donning of sterile gloves, use of sterile consumables and media are basic requirements. Clean disposable (but non-sterilised) gloves may be used as this will be cheaper but the gloves should not touch the inside of the sterile containers or the semen sample. It is well advised to carry out all work under a laminar flow hood. Two commonly used sperm preparation methods will now be described. Preliminary steps include measuring the volume of semen in each pot of the split ejaculate with a sterile graduated pipette. Carry out semen analysis as described in the previous section. It is not necessary to repeat a stained morphology assessment provided it was carried out recently. A quick morphological assessment on an unstained wet preparation is performed this time. Label sterile 5 ml or 13 ml conical centrifuge tubes with patient identifying information. Working with small volumes of semen (1–2 ml) in several tubes is more efficient than using a large volume of semen in a single tube. The particular culture medium used for sperm preparation depends on factors such as individual preference, easy availability and cost considerations. In-house manufacture of culture medium is probably not cost-effective in an IUI programme and it may be difficult to ensure maintenance of the highest standards in quality. The choice really lies between buying a ready to use medium such as Gamete–100 (Scandinavian IVF Science AB, Gothenburg, Sweden) or a physiological solution such as Earle's balanced salt solution (EBSS) and adding a protein source, antibiotics and energy substrates to it as described below. The reader should be conscious of the fact that assisted reproduction technology has evolved to a stage where it is becoming ethically and legally unacceptable to continue using materials not specifically manufactured for human use. Care should be taken to ensure that culture media is of pharmaceutical grade and meant for culture of human gametes and embryos. Alternative culture media can be used in the following sections where EBSS is mentioned.

## Preparation of supplemented Earle's balanced salt solution (EBSS)

### Required materials

500 ml bottle of EBSS
Pyruvic acid
600 mg crystalline penicillin
20% (w/v) human serum albumin
Millipore filter
Sterile test tubes
Syringes (1 and 5 ml)
Graduated pipette (25 ml)
Sterile 50 ml conical flasks

*Procedure*

1. Aliquot 5 ml of EBSS into a test tube.
2. Measure out 55 mg of pyruvate and add to the fluid in the test tube. Use a vortex mixer to ensure that it dissolves completely.
3. Draw up this solution with the syringe, attach a millipore syringe filter and deposit the filtered solution into the 500 ml bottle of EBSS.
4. Dissolve the penicillin powder in 5 ml of sterile tissue culture-quality distilled water. Withdraw 0.32 ml of the penicillin solution and add to the 500 ml bottle of EBSS.
5. Recap the bottle of EBSS and invert to mix.
6. Decant about 2 ml from this prepared solution and check the osmolarity with an osmometer to confirm that it lies between 284 and 288 mOsm/kg
7. Aliquot into 10 sterile 50 ml flasks.
8. Label and date these flasks and store in the refrigerator until required.
9. Before use add 0.8 ml of 20% human serum albumin to the flask. Label and place the flask in a humidified $CO_2$ incubator to equilibrate overnight. Please note that the cap has to be loosened to allow percolation of the gas mixture through the contents of the flask.

### Wash and swim-up method (Figure 8.3)

1. Place 1 ml of semen in a centrifuge tube.
2. Add 4 ml of culture medium to this volume of semen and mix thoroughly by drawing the sample in and out of a plastic pipette.
3. Centrifuge at 500 $g$ for 10 minutes and discard the supernatant.
4. Resuspend the pellet in another 4 ml of culture medium.
5. Centrifuge at 250 $g$ for 5 minutes and discard the supernatant.
6. Very carefully layer 1 ml of culture medium onto the pellet, taking care not to disturb it.
7. Place the tube in a slanting position (45 degrees) and incubate at 37 °C for 1 hour.
8. Carefully remove the top 500 µl of medium and place it in a clean tube, mixing it well.
9. Assess the sperm density and motility, as detailed above.

Step 6 may be modified in the following way to improve the recovery of motile spermatozoa: Resuspend the pellet in 300 µl of culture medium and gently place this in the bottom of a tube containing another 500 µl of culture medium as depicted in Figure 8.4.

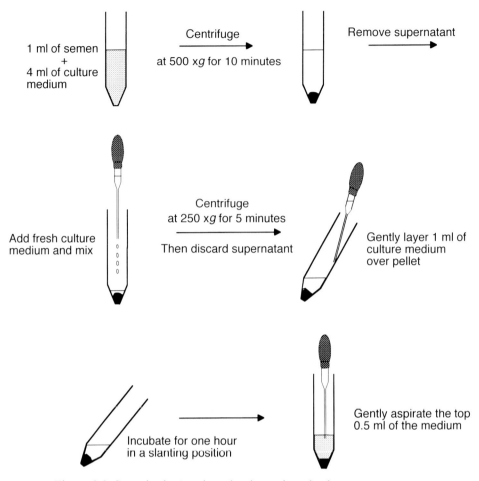

Figure 8.3. Steps in the 'wash and swim-up' method.

## Use of density gradient centrifugation media

Reactive oxygen species cause lipid peroxidation of the sperm membrane, thereby leading to a loss of motility and decreased fertilising ability (Aitken *et al.* 1989, 1991). While normal spermatozoa do produce small amounts of these superoxide radicals, production is many times more in dead or defective spermatozoa and white blood cells found in the ejaculate (Ford 1990). In view of this, it is important to separate normal motile spermatozoa from these noxious constituents of the ejaculate at the outset of the preparation process. Incorporation of centrifugation of the semen sample through bouyant density media as the first step in the sperm preparation technique fulfils this requirement and avoids or significantly decreases the collection of these unwanted cells and debris in the pellet that forms at the bottom of the centrifuge tube.

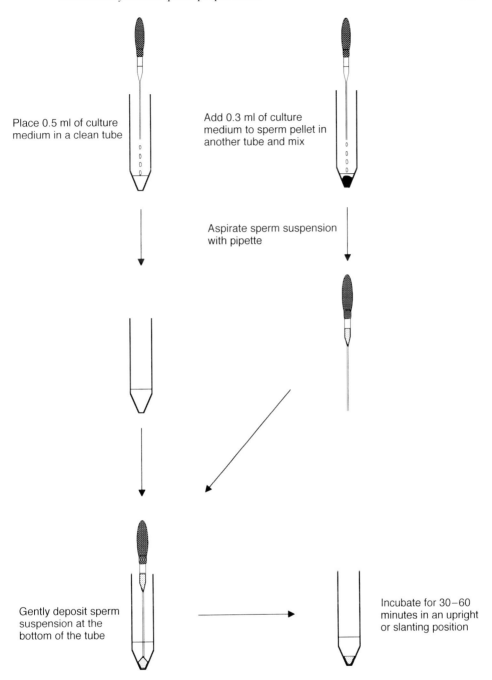

Figure 8.4. An alternative method for placing a sperm suspension under fresh culture medium for 'swim-up'.

For many years, Percoll (Pharmacia LKB Biotechnology, Uppsala, Sweden) was the most commonly used density gradient centrifugation medium for sperm preparation. It is a colloidal suspension of silica particles which are coated with polyvinyl pyrrolidone. A higher return of motile spermatozoa which score better at the zona-free hamster oocyte penetration test has been demonstrated in samples prepared with Percoll when compared with those prepared with the washing and centrifugation method (Ford 1990). Other workers have reported similar findings (Berger *et al.* 1985). Another advantage of using Percoll is that the colloidal particles it contains provide buoyant density that helps cushion spermatozoa during centrifugation thereby minimising any disruptive effects on the sperm nuclear chromatin arrangement. It also enhances the percentage of spermatozoa with a normal morphology where the fresh ejaculate contains 5% or more normal forms (Fleming *et al.* 1994; Hall *et al.* 1995). Percoll has been marketed for use in research settings only but it somehow gained wide popularity in clinical assisted conception treatment programmes. A recent communication from the producer, however, has reiterated the fact that it is not meant for human use; any practitioner who still persists in using this compound thus may be liable to legal sanctions.

Rather fortuitously, two companies have just began marketing variants which they claim to be suitable for human use. PureSperm (NidaCon Laboratories AB, Gothenburg, Sweden) is an iso-osmotic solution containing silica particles coated with reactive silane. Scandinavian IVF Science AB (Gothenburg, Sweden) has the license to market a sperm preparation kit (PureSperm System) which consists of ampoules of PureSperm, diluent medium and sperm washing medium. All materials used in their manufacture are of pharmaceutical grade quality and the contents of the ampoules are sterile. While Percoll commonly has endotoxin levels of between 25 and 50 EU/ml, much lower levels of 2–4 EU/ml are found in PureSperm. The manufacturers of the latter product are presently working towards further reduction of the endotoxin levels to below the level of 0.125 EU/mL stipulated for injectables and infusion products by the Food and Drug Administration in the USA (P. Holmes; personal communication). Irvine Scientific (Santa Ana, USA) produces and markets ISolate sperm preparation medium which is also an iso-osmotic colloidal suspension of silica particles coated with silane. Either PureSperm or ISolate can be used for sperm preparation as described in the following sections. Only PureSperm is mentioned for ease of narration.

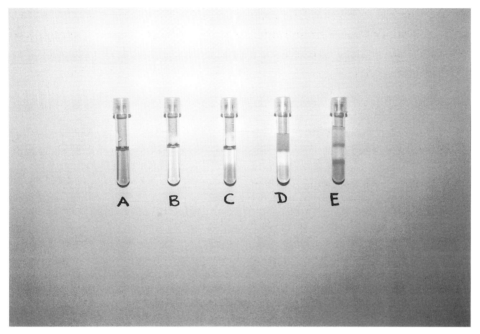

Figure 8.5. Use of PureSperm for sperm preparation. (A) 90% PureSperm; (B) 45% PureSperm; (C) 90% PureSperm carefully overlaid with 45% PureSperm; (D) discontinuous gradient of 45/90% PureSperm overlaid with semen sample; and (E) appearances following centrifugation: much of the debris is trapped at the interface between the 45% and 90% PureSperm layers. Normal motile spermatozoa pass through the PureSperm layers, during centrifugation, to form a pellet at the bottom of the tube.

### Required materials

100% (w/v) PureSperm
Supplemented EBSS or any other gamete preparation medium such as Gamete-100 (Scandinavian IVF Science AB, Gothenburg, Sweden)
Conical base centrifuge tubes
Pasteur pipettes and rubber bung
Graduated pipettes (5 and 10 ml)

### Dilution of PureSperm

Various workers have used different concentrations of Percoll but a discontinuous 45–90% Percoll gradient achieves satisfactory separation of live motile and normal spermatozoa from other constituents of semen (Fleming *et al.* 1994). The manufacturers of PureSperm and ISolate have also suggested the use of a similar concentration gradient. The stock solution of 100% PureSperm is diluted with culture medium in a ratio of 9:1 in order to obtain the 90% solution. An aliquot of the 90% solution is then diluted with an equal volume of culture medium to produce the 45% solution. The following exercise serves to illustrate this:

- To prepare 10 ml of 90% PureSperm or ISolate solution add 1 ml of culture medium to 9 ml of 100% PureSperm or ISolate solution.
- To prepare 10 ml of 45% PureSperm or ISolate solution make a 90% solution as described above. Then take 5 ml from the 90% solution and mix it with 5 ml of culture medium. Alternatively, mix 4.5 ml of PureSperm with 5.5 ml of culture medium to get 10 ml of the 45% solution.

The volume of 45% and 90% PureSperm solutions to be prepared depends on the laboratory workload and is best carried out at least a day before use. At the end of each working day unused prepared PureSperm is returned to the fridge and brought out the next morning to warm up to room temperature on the bench. Alternatively, PureSperm solutions are prepared at the end of each working day and left at room temperature overnight to ensure they are at the right temperature first thing in the morning, especially if sperm preparation routinely starts early in the day.

Two sperm preparation methods that involve the use of PureSperm will now be described. In the first technique the pellet of washed spermatozoa is resuspended in an aliquot of culture medium while in the second method, a final stage for swim-up of motile spermatozoa is incorporated. The decision on which method to use depends on operator experience, needs and the quality of the semen sample. We recommend inclusion of the swim-up step as this results in further separation of motile from immotile sperm that were not trapped in the PureSperm gradients.

### Semen preparation with PureSperm (Figures 8.5 and 8.6)

#### Without swim-up

1. Add 1 ml of 90% PureSperm solution into the centrifuge tube using a Pasteur pipette.
2. With another pipette GENTLY layer 1 ml of 45% PureSperm over the 90% solution in the tube. Take care to avoid mixing of the two solutions.
3. Overlay 1 ml of semen onto the PureSperm gradients in the tube.
4. Transfer the tube to the bench centrifuge and spin at 500 $g$ for 10 minutes.
5. Slowly pass a Pasteur pipette through the layers of PureSperm while squeezing gently on the rubber bung so that an air bubble is present at the tip of the pipette to prevent any debris entering the pipette until it gets to the bottom of

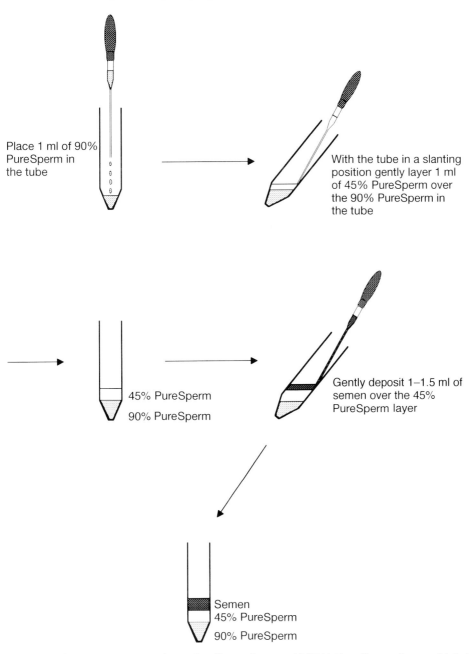

Figure 8.6. Preparation of a discontinuous 45/90% PureSperm layer which is then overlaid with semen ready for centrifugation.

the tube. Use it in aspirating the bottom 0.25 ml of PureSperm suspension containing the motile spermatozoa which is then transferred to a fresh tube. An alternative method is to rapidly pass a Pasteur pipette through the layers of PureSperm to the bottom of the tube to allow minimal time for any contaminating debris in the upper layer of PureSperm to enter the pipette.

6. Add 2 ml of culture medium and mix. Centrifuge at 250 g for 5 minutes.
7. Carefully remove the supernatant so as not to disturb the sperm pellet, leaving about 50 μl at the bottom of the tube. Add 1 ml of culture medium, mix gently and centrifuge at 250 g for another 5 minutes.
8. Gently remove the supernatant leaving about 50 μl at the bottom of the tube.
9. The volume of culture medium to add at this stage depends on the required inseminating volume. If the volume is to be 300 μl, add 250 μl of fresh culture medium. If fallopian tube sperm perfusion (see Chapter 9) is to be carried out, the sperm pellet is resuspended in 4 ml of culture medium.
10. Examine a drop from this tube under the microscope and record the concentration of sperm, motility, progression and morphology.
11. Place the sperm preparation into an incubator maintained at 37 °C until needed.

*With swim-up step*

The procedure is the same with that described above up to Step 8; then:

9. Very carefully layer 500 μl of culture medium onto the pellet, taking care not to disturb it. Alternatively resuspend the pellet in about 200 μl of culture medium, aspirate into the Pasteur pipette and carefully deposit at the bottom of a test tube containing 500 μl of culture medium.
10. Place the capped tube, slightly tilted to one side at an angle of 45 degrees, in a test tube rack in the incubator for 30–60 minutes to allow motile sperm to swim up to the upper layers.
11. Carefully bring the tube back to an upright position and aspirate the top 250 μl of the fluid in the tube and place in a fresh labelled tube. Make this up to 4 ml if fallopian tube sperm perfusion is to be performed.
12. Examine a drop from this tube under the microscope and record the concentration of sperm, their motility, progression and morphology.
13. Place the sperm preparation in an incubator maintained at 37 °C until needed.

**References**

Aitken R. J., Clarkson J. S., Hargreave T. B., Irvine D. S. & Wu F. C. (1989) Analysis of the relationship between defective sperm function and the generation of reactive oxygen species in cases of oligozoospermia. *Journal of Andrology* **10**, 214–220.

Aitken R. J., Irvine D. S. & Wu F. C. (1991) Prospective analysis of sperm–oocyte fusion and reactive oxygen species generation as criteria for the diagnosis of infertility. *American Journal of Obstetrics and Gynecology* **164**, 542–552.

Berger T., Marrs R. P. & Moyer D. L. (1985) Comparison of techniques for selection of motile spermatozoa. *Fertility and Sterility* **43**, 268–273.

Farris E. J. & Murphy D. P. (1960) The characteristics of the two parts of the partitioned ejaculation and the advantages of its use for intrauterine insemination. *Fertility and Sterility* **11**, 465–469.

Fleming S., Green S., Hall J. & Fishel S. (1994) Sperm function and its manipulation for microassisted fertilisation. *Baillière's Clinical Obstetrics and Gynaecology* **8**, 43–64.

Ford W. C. L. (1990) The role of oxygen free radicals in the pathology of human spermatozoa: implications for IVF. In: *Clinical IVF Forum.* (P. L. Matson, B. A. Lieberman, eds), Manchester University Press, Manchester, pp.123–139.

Hall J., Fishel S. B. & Timson J. (1993) Evaluation of sperm morphology in relation to conventional in vitro fertilization (IVF) and micro-assisted fertilization (MAF). *Human Reproduction* (supplement), **8**, 90.

Hall J., Fishel S. B., Timson J. A., Dowell K. & Klentzeris L. D. (1995) Human sperm morphology evaluation pre- and post-Percoll gradient centrifugation. *Human Reproduction* **10**, 342–346.

Kruger T. F., Ackerman S. B., Simmons K. F., Swanson R. J., Brugo S. S. & Acosta A. A. (1987) A quick reliable staining technique for human sperm morphology. *Archives of Andrology* **18**, 275–277.

MacLeod J. & Hotchkiss R. S. (1942) Distribution of spermatozoa and of certain chemical constituents in human ejaculate. *Journal of Urology* **48**, 225–229.

Menkveld R., Stander F. S. H., Kotze T. J., Kruger T. F. & van Zyl J. A. (1990) The evaluation of morphological characteristics of human spermatozoa according to stricter criteria. *Human Reproduction* **5**, 586–592.

Mortimer D. (1994) Sperm washing. In: *Practical Laboratory Andrology.* Oxford University Press, New York. pp. 267–286.

Oehninger S. & Kruger T. (1995) The diagnosis of male infertility by semen quality: clinical significance of sperm morphology assessment. *Human Reproduction* **10**, 1037–1038.

Perez-Pelaez M. & Cohen M. R. (1965) The split ejaculate in homologous insemination. *International Journal of Fertility* **10**, 25–30.

Van der Ven H., Bhattacharyya A. K., Binor Z., Leto S. & Zaneveld L. J. D. (1982) Inhibition of human sperm capacitation by a high molecular weight factor from human seminal plasma. *Fertility and Sterility* **38**, 753–755.

World Health Organization (1992) *WHO laboratory manual for the examination of human semen and sperm-cervical mucus interaction,* third edition. Cambridge University Press, Cambridge.

# 9
# Intrauterine insemination techniques

GODWIN I. MENIRU and PETER R. BRINSDEN

**Theoretical considerations**

Artificial insemination may be carried out by intravaginal, peri-cervical or intracervical deposition of neat semen or intrauterine insemination (IUI) of prepared sperm samples. It is only with IUI, however, that one is assured of spermatozoa reaching the uterine cavity in predetermined numbers. The other three methods suffer from the disadvantage of requiring receptive cervical mucus for optimal passage of spermatozoa through the cervical canal and into the uterine cavity; even then, it is not possible to predict the proportion of inseminated sperm that will reach the uterine cavity. Published evidence supports IUI as being superior to intracervical insemination in situations of reduced sperm concentration and motility, cervical hostility and antisperm antibodies (Martinez *et al*. 1993). This superiority is also evident when donor semen is used (Wainer *et al*. 1995). Intratubal and direct intraperitoneal insemination are other methods of artificial insemination, but they are more invasive and have a higher risk of complications.

Following IUI, part of the inseminated fluid may track backwards and spermatozoa lodge in crypts of the cervical canal (Ripps *et al*. 1994). They subsequently reappear at intervals to ascend the upper genital tract thereby maintaining a continuous supply of motile spermatozoa to the fallopian tubes. The quality of ejaculated or washed sperm affects their survival after IUI. Hence poor samples may need to be inseminated more frequently or closer to the time of predicted ovulation. The fallopian tubes may be perfused at the time of IUI or spermatozoa may reach there later on from their site of deposition in the uterine cavity. Junior *et al*. (1992) determined that insemination volumes of 0.4 ml or more reached the fallopian tubes. Variation in the capacity and distensibility of the uterine cavity may however affect the extent of tubal perfusion in individual cases. Furthermore, the normal insemination

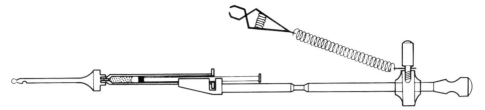

Figure 9.1. Drawing of the Makler Insemination Device, showing an insemination cannula attached to a tuberculin syringe which is mounted on a carrier.

catheter may not achieve a good seal at the cervical os thereby leading to reflux of the inseminated fluid during the injection process. These factors could be partly responsible for the present lack of consensus on optimal number and timing of inseminations in each cycle of treatment (Brook *et al.* 1994; Ransom *et al.* 1994; Khalifa *et al.* 1995).

Insemination should be carried out using aseptic techniques to avoid causing genital tract infection. The procedure must be gentle and atraumatic as products of local tissue reaction to injury may be hostile to spermatozoa and impede fertilisation. A soft pliable catheter such as the Wallace insemination catheter (H. G. Wallace Ltd, Colchester, UK) may be used for IUI. It has a slightly firmer outer sleeve which may be advanced first to cannulate the cervical canal before sliding forward the softer catheter inside it. In more difficult cases, slight traction on the cervix with the aid of a single tooth vulsellum usually straightens out the angle between the uterine cavity and cervical canal. Application of the vulsellum causes discomfort which however is often transient. Asking the patient to cough at the time of application of the instrument serves to distract her attention and produce a counter stimulus. A firmer catheter such as the Frydman catheter (CCD Laboratories, Paris, France) may be used when this fails. The patient lies supine or in a Trendelenburg position after insemination and this is aimed at ensuring dispersion of fluid in the uterine cavity and upwards through the fallopian tubes before ambulation.

Makler *et al.* (1984) described a device for injecting and retaining small volumes of prepared sperm suspension in the uterine cavity and cervical canal (Figures 9.1 and 9.2). This equipment is now being manufactured by Sefi-Medical Instruments, Haifa, Israel, and consists of a semi-rigid cannula that can be fitted on a 1 ml tuberculin syringe. A carrier system serves to hold the syringe in place and maintain firm contact between the base of the cannula and the cervix thereby preventing leakage of injected fluid. Two cannula sizes are available (Figures 9.3 and 9.4). The short type (15 mm long) is used for intracervical insemination while the longer type (50 mm in length) is for IUI. These

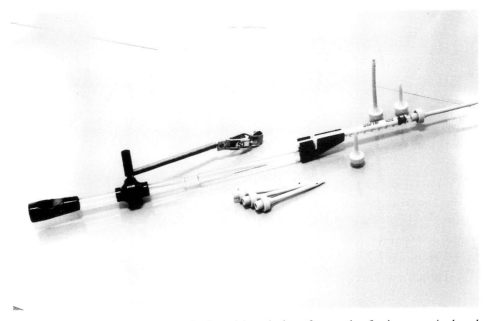

Figure 9.2. The Makler device with a choice of cannulae for intracervical and intrauterine insemination.

workers reported good tolerance of this device by patients and 12 pregnancies in a group of 47 treated couples (26%).

How much of an advantage, if any, is conferred by flooding the tubes with larger volumes of fluid and high concentrations of spermatozoa? It is clearly not physiological as animal studies and preliminary evidence from experiments in humans have shown that spermatozoa in the fallopian tubes rarely exceed a few hundred in number at any point in time after copulation. The uterine cavity and fallopian tubes have at most, a filmy coating of transudated fluid under normal conditions. There is a theoretical chance that forced flow of a large inseminating volume of fluid may sweep back into the peritoneal cavity any oocyte that has already been successfully picked up by the fallopian tubes. The immunological consequences of presenting such a large antigenic load of spermatozoa and possibly other foreign cells and cellular debris to the peritoneal cavity are not known with certainty at present. Kremer (1979) found that IUI led to a significant increase in the titre of serum antisperm antibodies in women already known to have these antibodies.

Despite the aforementioned uncertainties, a number of techniques have been developed in recent years for irrigating the fallopian tubes with prepared sperm suspension and depositing part of this fluid in the pouch of Douglas. Proponents believe that these methods provide a more effective concentration

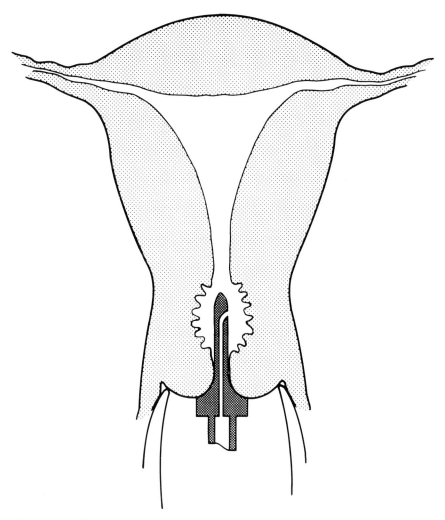

Figure 9.3. The short Makler cannula positioned for intracervical insemination.

of spermatozoa around the oocyte as well as treating partial tubal obstruction caused by thick viscid mucus or polyps. One group of techniques is based on catheterisation of the fallopian tube under laparoscopic, ultrasound or tactile guidance (Berger 1987; Jansen et al. 1988; Lucena et al. 1989; Pratt et al. 1991) but potential complications of trauma, infection and vasovagal shock limit their usefulness. They make IUI more invasive and technically demanding thereby undermining its major attribute of simplicity. The second group of methods dispenses with tubal catheterisation, but achieves similar effects, with slow injection of 4 ml of a sperm suspension through the cervical canal. This so-called fallopian tube sperm perfusion suffered initially from the drawback

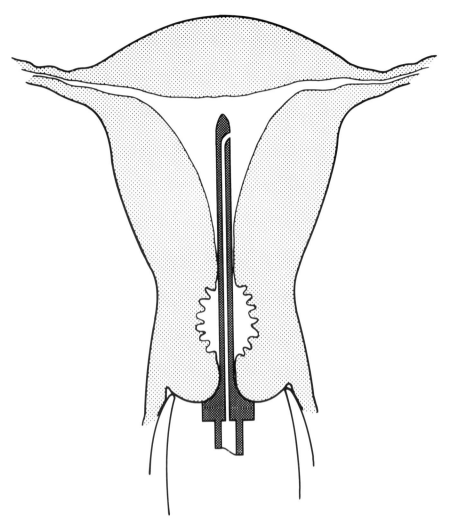

Figure 9.4. The long Makler cannula in the usual position for intrauterine insemination.

of fluid reflux due to the lack of a proper sealing device at the cervical os. A number of measures have been proposed to prevent this reflux, such as the application of a clamp on the cervix or the use of a paediatric Foley's catheter (Li 1993). The latter device is passed into the uterine cavity and the balloon inflated so as to occlude the junction between the uterine cavity and the cervical canal. The Fallopian Sperm Transfer System (FAST® System; CCD Laboratories, Paris, France) is another device for overcoming this problem of fluid reflux. Fanchin *et al.* (1995a) recently reported a significantly higher clinical pregnancy rate of 40%, per cycle of treatment, associated with use of the

FAST® System, compared with 20% in women who had conventional IUI of 0.2 ml of sperm suspension. That study was based on patients who had normal semen parameters on analysis. This same group of workers subsequently reported fallopian tube sperm perfusion to be even more efficacious than conventional IUI in patients with moderate abnormalities of semen parameters (Fanchin *et al.* 1995b). Not all workers, however, have shown superiority of fallopian tube sperm perfusion. Karande *et al.* (1995) found a similar overall pregnancy rate of 10.8% in women who had conventional IUI and those who were inseminated with fallopian tube sperm perfusion. These two studies differed in a number of areas, which included study design, patient population, treatment protocols and sperm preparation. Further studies are needed to confirm or refute the usefulness of this method of insemination.

## Insemination techniques

The prepared sperm sample is collected from the laboratory after confirming it and the patient's identity by reference to the laboratory request form and the hospital notes. Identity of the sample is further cross-checked by the semenologist, the couple and the clinician. The sample is maintained at 37 °C in a tube warmer or held in a fist. It can, however, be left at normal room temperature but this should not be for long periods. Usually, few instruments are needed for this procedure (Figure 9.5) which is ideally carried out in the theatre (Figure 9.6) or a similarly equipped room. Although the clinician does not need to put on sterile operating gowns he should wear a cap and mask and wash his hands and forearms with antiseptic detergent. This is followed by thorough rinsing with clean water, drying with sterile paper towels and donning sterile powder-free gloves. The patient is placed in the lithotomy position, but the dorsal position with flexion of the hip and knees and some abduction of the hip will suffice, provided the exposure is satisfactory. The vulva is cleansed with warm normal saline and sterile drapes put in place. After moistening a Cusco's speculum with normal saline it is inserted gently into the vagina to expose the cervix, which is then wiped gently with cotton wool balls soaked in normal saline. Subsequent manoeuvres depend on the particular technique of insemination being used.

### *Conventional technique*

An insemination catheter is attached to a 1 ml syringe and used in drawing up the prepared sperm sample. It is important that the volume of the sample is standardised and in our practice is usually 0.3 ml, although we have recently

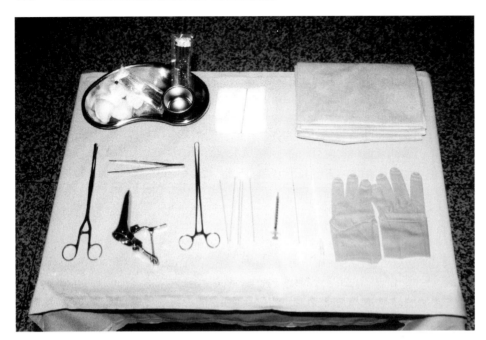

Figure 9.5. Instruments laid out for intrauterine insemination.

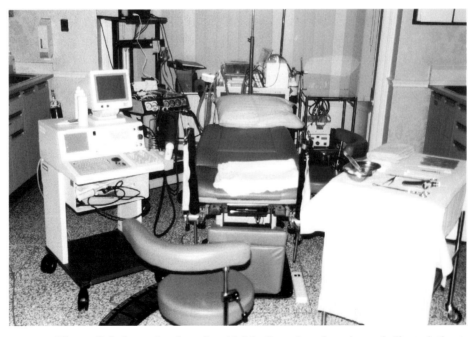

Figure 9.6. Insemination should ideally take place in a dedicated theatre although other venues may be acceptable.

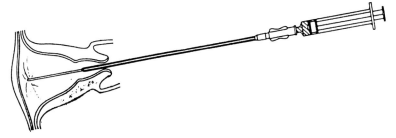

Figure 9.7. Intrauterine insemination with a conventional catheter. The insemination volume has to be kept low to prevent back flow and loss of a significant volume of the sperm suspension into the vagina.

begun evaluating an insemination volume of 1 ml. It should be appreciated that the dead space in a catheter is significant when compared to the insemination volume of the sperm suspension. For example, one of the Frydman catheters has a dead space of about 0.53 ml. If the syringe is loaded with the sperm suspension before attaching the catheter, no fluid will be ejected into the uterine cavity when the plunger is depressed. The best way of avoiding this problem is to first attach the catheter to the syringe and use it in aspirating the sample from the test tube into the proximal part of the catheter. This will eliminate the dead space.

The cannula is passed through the cervical canal and into the uterine cavity for a distance of about 6 cm and the plunger depressed slowly to expel the fluid (Figure 9.7). During injection, this air column now returns to its former location in the catheter and in the process displaces the fluid out of the catheter tip. The cannula and speculum are withdrawn and the patient lies supine for 5–10 minutes before getting up. If the couch is equipped with relevant controls, it can be used to raise the patient's hips slightly so as to prevent backflow of the inseminated fluid through the external os and aid its spread into the fallopian tubes.

### Using the Makler insemination device

The appropriate cannula is attached to the syringe which is then used in aspirating 0.2 ml of the sperm suspension. Following this, the syringe is mounted on the tip of the carrier. The cannula is gently inserted into the cervical canal (short cannula) or the uterine cavity (long cannula) until the flared base of the cannula fits the external os snugly. The clamp is next fixed to the speculum as shown in Figure 9.8 and tension in the spring adjusted so as to maintain the base of the cannula in firm apposition to the cervical os. The plunger of the

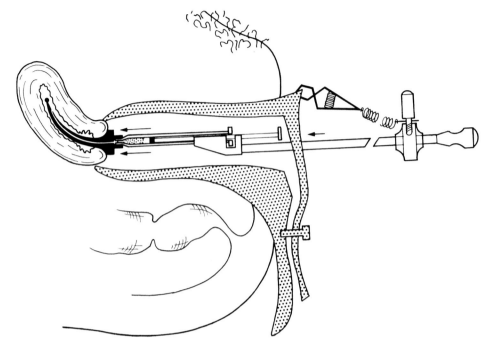

Figure 9.8. Intrauterine insemination with the Makler device. The cannula is held firmly in apposition to the cervix by means of a spring-loaded clip that is attached to the vaginal speculum.

syringe is slowly depressed to inject the sperm preparation. The instrument is removed after 10–20 minutes and the patient allowed home.

### *Using the Fallopian Sperm Transfer System (Fanchin et al. 1995a)*

The single use FAST® System is made up of essentially two sections (Figures 9.9–9.11). The rigid injection catheter ends in an acorn tip, while the vacuum catheter has a more pliable cup that is available in two sizes of 30 and 35 mm diameter. The technique of insemination has to take into consideration the fact that this injection catheter has a dead space of about 1.5 ml. The 5 ml syringe is attached to the injection catheter, which is then used to draw up the 4 ml of sperm suspension. About 1.5 ml of air will be seen in the syringe. Care should be taken to ensure that this is the last to be injected during the insemination procedure so that it displaces the sperm suspension from the dead space of the catheter.

The acorn tip is placed at the external os followed by the vacuum cup which encircles the cervix. The plunger of the 20 ml syringe is pulled backwards thereby creating a vacuum in the cup which serves to hold the injection catheter

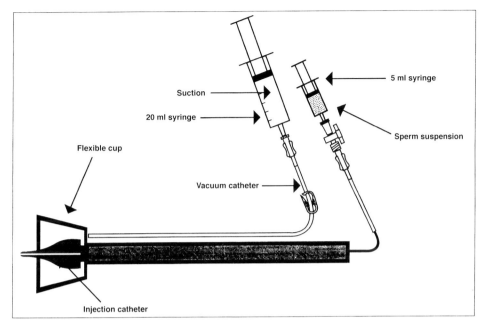

Figure 9.9. Components of the FAST® System (From Fanchin, R., Olivennes, F., Righini, C., Hazout, A., Schwab, B. & Frydman, R. A new system for fallopian tube sperm perfusion leads to pregnancy rates twice as high as standard intrauterine insemination. *Fertility and Sterility* 1995; 64, 505–510). Reproduced with permission of the publisher, the American Society for Reproductive Medicine (The American Fertility Society).

tip in firm apposition to the external os. The locking device is closed when a satisfactory vacuum has been obtained. The sperm suspension is then injected over 2 minutes, followed by release of the vacuum and withdrawal of the FAST® System. The patient rests for a few minutes on the couch before getting up.

There is no agreement at present on the optimal number of inseminations to be performed in each cycle of treatment with the FAST® System. Fanchin *et al.* (1995a) carried out only one timed insemination while Karande *et al.* (1995) inseminated the patients on 2 consecutive days.

### Post-insemination instructions

Patients are provided with laboratory request forms for pregnancy tests which are performed 14 days after the first insemination. The most accurate tests are based on detection of the beta subunit of human chorionic gonadotrophin in a blood sample. More specific instructions depend on the type of protocol for

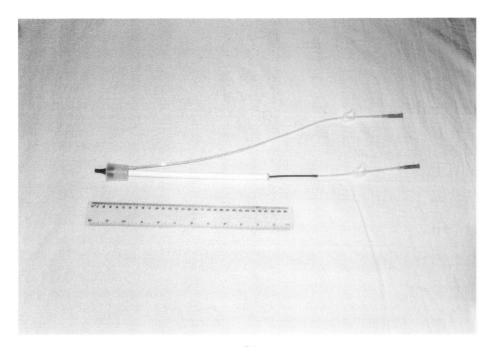

Figure 9.10. An assembled FAST® System.

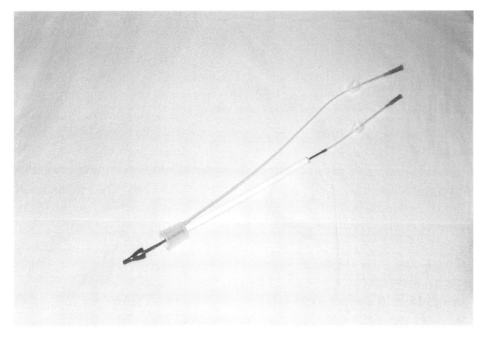

Figure 9.11. The FAST® System with the vacuum cup drawn back to show the acorn-shaped tip of the injection catheter.

ovarian stimulation that was used. If for example, gonadotrophin releasing hormone agonists were used, progesterone should be administered until a negative pregnancy test result is obtained, or until the 12th week of gestation in those who become pregnant. Arrangements should be made to see the couple irrespective of the outcome of the treatment cycle. Those who become pregnant will have confirmatory ultrasound scans and subsequent referral for antenatal care, while those who fail to achieve a pregnancy will have discussions on further management options.

### Acknowledgements

Figures 9.1–9.4 and 9.7 were kindly supplied by Sefi-Medical Instruments, Haifa, Israel.

### References

Berger G. S. (1987) Intratubal insemination. *Fertility and Sterility* **48**, 328–330.

Brook P. F., Barratt C. L. R. & Cooke I. D. (1994) The more accurate timing of insemination with regard to ovulation does not create a significant improvement in pregnancy rates in a donor insemination program. *Fertility and Sterility* **61**, 308–313.

Fanchin R., Olivennes F., Righini C., Hazout A., Schwab B. & Frydman R. (1995a) A new system for fallopian tube sperm perfusion leads to pregnancy rates twice as high as standard intrauterine insemination. *Fertility and Sterility* **64**, 505–510.

Fanchin R., Olivennes F., Righini C., Hazout A., Fernandez H., Schwab B., Selva J. & Frydman R. (1995b) A new system for fallopian tube sperm perfusion leads to pregnancy rates three times as high as standard IUI in cases of sperm abnormalities. *15th World Congress on Fertility and Sterility,* Montpellier, France, 17–22 September 1995.

Jansen R. P. S., Anderson J. C., Radonic I., Smit J. & Sutherland P. D. (1988) Pregnancies after ultrasound-guided fallopian insemination with cryostored donor semen. *Fertility and Sterility* **49**, 920–922.

Junior J. G. F., Baruffi R. L. R., Mauri A. L. & Stone S. C. (1992) Radiological evaluation of incremental intrauterine instillation of contrast material. *Fertility and Sterility* **58**, 1065–1067.

Karande V. C., Rao R., Pratt D. E., Balin M., Levrant S., Morris R., Dudkeiwicz A. & Gleicher N. (1995) A randomized prospective comparison between intrauterine insemination and fallopian sperm perfusion for the treatment of infertility. *Fertility and Sterility* **64**, 638–640.

Khalifa Y., Redgment C. J., Tsirigotis M., Grudzinskas J. G. & Craft I. L (1995) The value of single versus repeated insemination in intra-uterine donor insemination cycles. *Human Reproduction* **10**, 153–154.

Kremer J. (1979) A new technique for intrauterine insemination. *International Journal of Fertility* **24**, 53–56.

Li T. C. (1993) A simple, non-invasive method of fallopian tube sperm perfusion. *Human Reproduction* **8**, 1848–1850.

Lucena E., Ruiz J. A., Mendoza J. C., Ortiz J. A., Lucena C., Gomez M. & Arango

A. (1989) Vaginal intratubal insemination (VITI) and vaginal GIFT, endosonographic technique: early experience. *Human Reproduction* **4,** 658–662.

Makler A., DeCherney A. & Naftolin F. (1984) A device for injecting and retaining a small volume of concentrated spermatozoa in the uterine cavity and cervical canal. *Fertility and Sterility* **42,** 306–308.

Martinez A. R., Bernardus R. E., Vermeiden J. P. W. & Schoemaker J. (1993) Basic questions on intrauterine insemination: an update. *Obstetrical and Gynecological Survey* **48,** 811–828.

Pratt D. E., Bieber E., Barnes R., Shangold G., Vignovic E. & Schreiber J. (1991) Transvaginal intratubal insemination by tactile sensation: a preliminary report. *Fertility and Sterility* **56,** 984–986.

Ransom M. X., Corsan G., Blotner M. B., Kemmann E. & Bohrer M. (1994) Does increasing frequency of intrauterine insemination improve pregnancy rates significantly during superovulation cycles? *Fertility and Sterility* **61,** 303–307.

Ripps B. A., Minhas B. S., Carson S. A. & Buster J. E. (1994) Intrauterine insemination in fertile women delivers larger numbers of sperm to the peritoneal fluid than intracervical insemination. *Fertility and Sterility* **61,** 398–400.

Wainer R., Merlet F., Ducot B., Bailly M., Tribalat S. & Lombroso R. (1995) Prospective randomized comparison of intrauterine and intracervical insemination with donor spermatozoa. *Human Reproduction* **10,** 2919–2922.

# 10

# The role of the nurse in an insemination programme

FRANCES E. BYNOE

## Introduction

The nurse's role in an intrauterine insemination (IUI) programme is a multifaceted one (Figure 10.1) and depends a great deal on local circumstances although there are fundamental principles that hold true in all situations. The nurse is the most constant person in the unit and tends to be the most approachable. She is therefore closest to patients and cannot insulate herself completely from their emotional states especially during times of intense distress such as having a cycle cancelled and on receiving the news of a negative pregnancy test following IUI. This should be an important consideration during recruitment of nursing staff. Infertility nursing can be an emotionally exhausting field in which to work and a strong united nursing team is a major attribute to the unit. Nurses need to be emotionally aware and available to their colleagues' needs also.

## The many roles of nurses

### *Clinical role*

The nurse welcomes the couple to the unit, directs them to the consulting room and often sits in during part or the whole of the clinical session with the doctor. She lends support to the couple who may find her less intimidating than the doctor. Furthermore, her presence serves to introduce her to that particular couple's clinical history. She prepares the patients for clinical examination and may assist the doctor in explaining some aspects of their management or reiterating points raised earlier on during the session. The couple will in turn find it easier relating to her outside the consulting room as they know she is already aware of their problem. Dividends rapidly accrue when important pieces of information begin to be released by the couple in the more informal and relaxing atmosphere outside the consulting room.

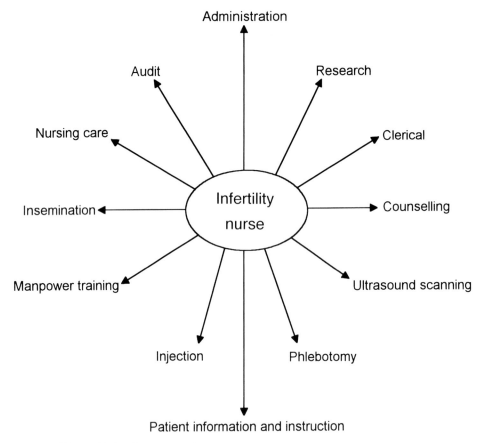

Figure 10.1. The many roles of an infertility nurse.

Nursing care continues during follicular stimulation. The nurse administers the required dose of gonadotrophin injections herself or teaches the patient how to self-inject at home. She withdraws blood from the patient for various tests required at any point during the infertility management. She usually sees the couple whenever they report to the centre for any aspect of their treatment. The nurse participates in daily meetings where patients' progress and response to treatment are discussed. She is also involved in scheduling appointments for ultrasound scans, insemination and blood tests.

### *Role in insemination*

The nurse prepares the instrument trolley before escorting the couple to the insemination room. The trolley is wiped down with 70% ethanol solution and not with other disinfectants which may leave residues that could be toxic to the spermatozoa. The woman is asked to remove her underwear and sit on the couch while her husband sits on a chair beside the couch. The nurse explains what is about to happen, who will be in the room and their role in the procedure. The doctor or nurse discusses the result of that day's semen analysis which is carried out on both the fresh and prepared sample. While waiting for the procedure to begin the nurse answers any questions the couple may have. She also tells them that specific post-procedural instructions will be given by the doctor. The patient is placed in the lithotomy position only when the doctor is ready to begin the insemination procedure.

In some units the nurse actually performs the insemination procedure herself. Just like in midwifery, anaesthesia, diabetic management, family planning and a host of other areas of patient care, nurses make effective practitioners when given such responsibilities. It is only the medico-legal requirements of the particular country that will determine how much autonomy the nurse can have. The key elements are proper training, supervision and support by the unit head with backup medical assistance being provided for difficult cases, who ideally should be identified before hand.

### *Counselling role*

All assisted conception treatment is fraught with emotion and stress. While IUI may be one of the least invasive treatments it still evokes great levels of stress. Couples have to be made as relaxed as possible. Infertility is a problem of the couple and not just one of them, therefore both the man and woman need to be involved and kept informed on the progress of treatment. The male partner should be encouraged, but not forced, to accompany his partner to the unit especially on the day(s) of insemination. The couple's need for information and reassurance is overwhelming although they generally tend to be well informed, having read many books and gathered much knowledge during the years of infertility. Time must however be spent with them in order to clarify any myths and misconceptions, answer any queries and provide encouragement.

The infertility nurse is not a counsellor, unless she has actually gone through a full course of theoretical and practical training. The nurse is however a very important part of the counselling process by virtue of her profile in the infertility unit. She bridges the gap between patient support commenced by the doctor at the initial consultation and the highly specialised and professional services of the counsellor. Specifically the nurse develops the ability to listen, observe, give support, provide information and acknowledge the couple's emotions and fears as being normal. The infertility nurse is equipped with counselling skills which she normally obtains through formal short-term courses or by experience and observing her colleagues.

### Administrative role

If an IUI service is being provided by a general or teaching hospital, it is likely that the nurse will be put in full charge of the section where this is being carried out while the consultants continue with their overall managerial activities in the Gynaecology Department. The nurse's administrative roles are diverse. She sees to the maintenance and smooth running of the service and ensures, among other things, that supplies are never exhausted before replenishing stocks.

### Conclusion

Versatility is the key word to be used when describing the role of the nurse in an IUI service. A broad-based education as well as experience will equip her towards handling responsibilities which may be thrust on her in the unit. The nurse will thrive and become a very important member of the unit when encouragement and support are given to her by the rest of the team.

# 11
# Principles and practice of semen cryopreservation

STEVEN GREEN and STEVEN D. FLEMING

### Historical perspective

The scientific history of semen cryopreservation really begins in 1677, with a letter from Antonie van Leeuwenhoek to the Royal Society of London, reporting his demonstration of motile cells in semen. Nearly 90 years passed before Jacobi in 1765 described an interest in the manipulation of gametes from his work with the external fertilisation of fish ova. This work is probably the earliest report of artificial insemination (AI). However it was a century after Leeuwenhoek's discovery when an Italian priest, the Abbe Lazzaro Spallanzani (1776), reported his observation that the spermatozoa of humans, stallion and frog could be cooled in snow for 30 minutes and re-warmed with recovery of movement. His studies encompassed both the foundations of semen cryopreservation and AI. Similarly, in 1897, Heape commented that over 50% of dog spermatozoa were still motile 18 hours after collection. Earlier in 1866, another Italian, Mantegazza, had reported his predictions that semen could be preserved by reducing the temperature. He wrote, 'If the human sperm can be preserved for more than 4 days at the temperature of melting ice without undergoing any change, then it is certain that scientists of the future will be able to improve breeds of horses and cattle without having to spend enormous sums of money in transporting thoroughbred stallions and bulls. It will be possible to carry out artificial insemination with frozen sperm sent rapidly from one locality to another. It should be feasible for a husband who dies on the battlefield to fertilise his wife and thus have legitimate sons even after his own death.' Today Mantegazza's predictions have largely been realised and his vision is even more remarkable in view of the lack of experimental evidence at the time.

The development of cryopreservation parallels the development of AI, and it was the potential commercial benefits of AI technology that spurred on the study of cryopreservation. The growing interest in the applications of AI led to investigations of the physical and chemical attributes of semen. Chang and Walton (1940) suggested that cooling extended the life of spermatozoa by a reduction in metabolic activity. The phenomenon of cold shock was first introduced in 1934 by Milovanov. Cold shock, or an acute sensitivity to cooling, is a phenomenon seen in some mammalian spermatozoa, particularly those of the ungulate species. Cold shock sensitivity has been correlated with the ratio of polyunsaturated to saturated phospholipids (Poulos *et al.* 1973; Darin-Bennett *et al.* 1974, 1977) and the proportion of cholesterol in the cell membrane (Darin-Bennett & White 1977). The causal effect of the cold shock phenomenon seems to be associated with phase changes affecting membrane function (Watson & Morris 1987). Egg yolk was introduced as a substance to protect spermatozoa against the effects of cold shock by Phillips in 1939. It is particularly the phospholipid component of the low density lipoprotein fraction that has been shown to protect the cell membrane from cold shock (Blackshaw 1954; Quinn *et al.* 1980; Watson 1981a). The nature of the protection afforded by egg yolk is not clearly understood although it appears to act at the plasma membrane surface (Watson 1981b), but induces no permanent alteration in membrane composition (Quinn *et al.* 1980). It does not influence the phase separation phenomenon (Holt & North 1984; De Leeuw *et al.* 1988), but it does prevent gross membrane disruption (Watson 1976). Egg yolk may therefore reduce the consequences of phase transition damage rather than totally prevent its occurrence. Egg yolk has been commonly incorporated into cryoprotectant diluents for this reason for many years. Fortunately, human spermatozoa are less sensitive to cold shock than many other mammalian species, and as there are cryoprotectant media formulations which do not contain egg yolk it is not an absolute requirement for successful human sperm cryopreservation (Mahadevan & Trounson 1983).

The early recognition of cold shock and the addition of egg yolk as a protective agent made possible the transport of bull semen at temperatures just above freezing (6–10 °C) for several days without loss of fertility. The commercial benefits resulting from this ability spurred on attempts to extend the viability of spermatozoa by reducing the temperature below freezing. Initial attempts, in 1940, of simply cooling the semen below freezing resulted in very poor recovery of spermatozoa as a consequence of ice crystal formation. The action of specific cryoprotective substances was not appreciated at this time and the earliest attempt to overcome ice crystal damage was to use vitrification, a process of cooling so rapidly that ice crystals did not form. Attempts to achieve vitrificaton were partially successful with sperm from frog, fowl and humans (Luyet & Hodapp 1938; Shaffner *et al.* 1941; Hoagland & Pincus 1942). The breakthrough in freeze preservation of spermatozoa occurred with the discovery that glycerol provided the conditions for survival of deep frozen fowl sperm (Polge *et al.* 1949). From this point, experiments in freeze preservation of spermatozoa became widespread and the first human babies from frozen semen were reported by Bunge *et al.* in 1954. The relatively recent development in human semen cryopreservation is due more to the changing climate of public opinion than to advances in technology. Historically, clinicians have preferred to use fresh semen rather than frozen-thawed semen in donor insemination programmes. Since 1986, it has been mandatory in the UK to use quarantined, cryopreserved semen to minimise the risk of infection due to the human immunodeficiency virus, the agent of acquired immune deficiency syndrome.

### The effect of cryopreservation on sperm membranes

Any process of sperm cryopreservation must result in the retention of motility and the ability of the spermatozoon, once the cell has been thawed, to penetrate and fuse with the oocyte. These are membrane function events. The various membranes of the spermatozoon such as the plasma membrane, and mitochondrial and acrosomal membranes, are unique aggregates of lipids and proteins assembled during spermatogenesis and modified during epididymal transit, storage and ejaculation (Hammerstedt & Parks 1987; Eddy 1988). Membrane function is determined by the interactions of the various components within the membrane, and any processing event that alters these interactions can be expected to alter function (Aloia *et al.* 1988). In a landmark paper in 1972, Singer and Nicolson proposed that cell membranes consisted of a mosaic structure of alternating globular integral proteins and a phospholipid bilayer (Figure 11.1). The mosaic structure was proposed to be a fluid in dynamic motion and was thought of as a two-dimensional orientated viscous solution. The concept of membrane structure, as one of a succession of layers where each layer has a unique lipid–protein distribution confirming relationships unique to a specific membrane function, would suggest that membranes could be susceptible to alterations during the freeze-thaw process. The protein–lipid interactions that occur within membranes are extremely important to cell function. Some lipids are preferentially clustered around integral membrane proteins (Quinn 1989) and we know that the lipid environment around a protein influences its functional properties (Carruthers & Melchior 1988a,b). When a biological membrane is cooled, a reorganisation of the membrane components is possible leading to aggregation of lipids that had been associated with membrane proteins. This would leave the proteins with alternate lipid partners (Quinn 1989). Rewarming would initially yield protein–lipid

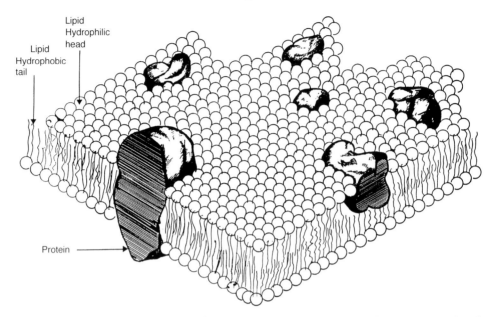

Figure 11.1. Diagrammatic representation of the mosaic structure of cell membranes, consisting of alternating globular integral proteins and a phospholipid bilayer. Adapted from Singer & Nicolson (1972).

partners different from those entering the freeze-thaw cycle. The original state, with its specific membrane properties would only be re-established where diffusion allowed reassembly of the components into their original display. As varying the temperature can affect the phase state of the membrane and alter its physical properties, it is extremely important to follow a cryopreservation protocol carefully.

The membrane bilayer may also be altered by a direct interaction with the cryoprotectant itself. As a reduction in temperature can alter membrane organisation caused by lipid reorganisation, this could alter the kinetics of water and cryoprotectant transport through the membrane (Mazur *et al.* 1974; Mazur & Miller 1976; Mazur & Rajotte 1981; De Gier 1989). With this in mind, one important consideration is whether to add glycerol to spermatozoa at 37 or 4 °C, as this would be expected to affect their ability to survive the freeze-thaw cycle and retain viability (Fiser & Fairfull 1989). For this reason glycerol is added to the cell at 37 °C, or more commonly at room temperature.

Dilution of spermatozoa in cryoprotectant containing 1 M glycerol can reduce cell volume to 50% of its isotonic state due to a rapid loss of intracellular water as a result of osmosis (Hammerstedt *et al.* 1978). A return to the original volume will occur over time as the glycerol enters the cell, but further shrinkage occurs on freezing as the extracellular water freezes. These events are reversed on thawing. It is not clear how the surface membranes of the spermatozoon accommodate these large changes in volume without folding or fusion. The nucleus occupies a major part of the sperm head and consists of highly condensed nucleoprotein and chromatin crosslinked with disulphide bridges (Bedford & Calvin 1974). Contraction of this structure would be limited. The acrosome and the intramembrane spaces in the anterior head may be able to accommodate some reduction in volume, but a substantial reduction in total volume of the spermatozoon could theoretically only be accommodated by the tail and midpiece regions. Studies with protoplasts have predicted that, on thawing, a lipid bilayer cannot expand more than 2–3% without rupture (Steponkus & Lynch 1989), but this is not the case with the spermatozoon when thawed and transfered into glycerol-free medium. It has been theorised that it may be possible that the midpiece and tail region are converted from a cylinder to a sphere, which has the highest volume to surface ratio of any geometrical shape (Hammerstedt *et al.* 1990). Thus a cylinder of fixed surface area would be able to accommodate a large volume expansion if the structure were converted to a sphere. Microscopic observations of a shape change involving a coiling of the tail within the membrane and a swelling of the midpiece towards a spherical shape have been observed in the bovine (Drevius & Erickson 1966; Bredderman & Foote 1969), the ram (Duncan 1988) and the human spermatozoa (Jeyendran *et al.* 1984).

Cryoprotectants can interact with the membrane and glycerol is known to alter the membrane bilayer (O'Leary & Levin 1984; Rudenko *et al.* 1984; Boggs & Rangaraj 1985). The response of each membrane type to the cryoprotectant could affect the permeability rates of water and ion movement, essential if the cell is going to survive the freeze-thaw process. Cryoprotectants can be metabolised by the cell, potentially creating an energy imbalance. Adenosine triphosphate (ATP) production is minimal in spermatozoa and ATP consumption is dominated by ion pumping and motility (Inskeep & Hammerstedt 1985). An increase in ATP consumption as a result of cryoprotectant metabolism could consequently result in an ATP deficit causing irreversible and degradative reactions within the cell (Hochachka 1986; Hochachka & Guppy 1987). The design of protocols for the cryopreservation of human spermatozoa demands an understanding of the spermatozoon as an integrated set of membrane-bound compartments, each having its own relationship with temperature, interaction with the cryoprotectant, and ATP requirements.

## Mode of action of cryoprotectants

Cryoprotectants are classified as permeating or non-permeating according to whether or not they enter the cell. In the absence of cryoprotective agents, very few spermatozoa of any species studied have been found to survive freezing to very low temperatures. Human spermatozoa are interesting in that none survive when thin films are plunged directly into liquid nitrogen, but some survival can be obtained if undiluted semen is cooled more slowly. Subjection of human spermatozoa to unprotected ultrarapid cooling in ampoules demonstrates that although most cells are damaged as a consequence of intracellular ice formation, some spermatozoa at the centre of the ampoule may survive. The initial cooling rate of the semen is probably retarded which could allow the formation of sufficient extracellular ice to reduce the amount of intracellular nucleation. Human sperm display considerable tolerance to solution effects, the increase in electrolytes caused by the formation and dissolution of ice during freezing and thawing, and no other species appears as hardy as the human. The addition of cryoprotective agents to semen greatly extends the tolerance of spermatozoa to freezing at slower rates, and the optimal cooling rate depends on the nature and concentration of the cryoprotectant used. The most commonly used agent for the cryoprotection of sperm is glycerol. The protective action of glycerol, a permeating agent, is due to its ability to reduce the concentration of electrolytes to which the cells are exposed during relatively slow cooling to eventual freezing. Cooling rates for the human spermatozoon, commonly around $-10$ °C per minute, are sufficient to permit extracellular crystallisation and consequent dehydration of the cell so that an ultrarapid drop to $-196$ °C, the temperature of liquid nitrogen, is not injurious, as sufficient water would have already been lost. Other agents added to some diluents are glycine and sucrose. Higher cryosurvival of spermatozoa has been observed when non-permeating agents such as sucrose are incorporated into the diluent (Watson 1979; Polge 1980). Sucrose, like other disaccharides, cannot penetrate cell membanes, but its presence in the extracellular medium exerts an osmotic protection regulating the rate of passage of water into and out of the cell. Mahadevan and Trounson reported in 1983 that the combination of 50 mM sucrose and 7.5% glycerol provided higher post-thaw motility than 7.5% glycerol alone.

## Cellular cryoinjury during the freeze-thaw cycle

It is now well established that for optimum cell survival the freezing rate must be matched with an appropriate thawing rate (Mazur 1984; Schneider 1986).

The cooling rate affects both the rate of water movement out of the cell and the extent of intracellular ice formation. The rate of freezing should be such that the extracellular ice forms at a rate to enable intracellular water to move out of the cell by osmosis without the intracellular water crystallising before dehydration of the cell is complete. Thus, when the spermatozoon arrives at $-196\,°C$ the intracellular and extracellular environment of the cell will be very different. Damage can still occur to the cell if the thaw rate is not compatible with the freeze rate. Too rapid a thaw can result in unbalanced rates of egress of cryoprotectant and influx of water, driven in turn by the rapid loss of the extracellular solid phase. If the thaw rate is too slow recrystallisation of microcrystals of intracellular water can result in damage to cellular organelles. The optimal warming rate depends on the cooling rate and is that which minimises damage due to inappropriate rates of solute and water transport across the membrane, and intracellular microcrystal formation.

## Equipment and materials used for semen cryopreservation

The process of semen cryopreservation comprises four stages: (1) preparative procedures, including semen collection, preparation of cryoprotectant diluent and dilution of the semen, (2) packaging of the semen-diluent mixture into freezing receptacles, (3) the freezing procedure itself, and (4) the storage of the cryopreserved material. Each step requires specific equipment and materials, and certain suppliers in the UK have kindly agreed for their products to be included in this chapter. Readers outside the UK can procure this equipment either from subsidiary companies or alternative sources in their locality.

### *Semen collection*

At the Nottingham University Research and Treatment Unit in Reproduction (NURTURE), semen is collected directly into specimen jars (L.I.P. Equipment & Services Ltd, Shipley, UK) (Figure 11.2); however, a number of patients have found these containers too small and an alternative is to use the semen collection equipment from Rocket Medical (Watford, UK) (Figure 11.3). These consist of funnel-shaped collectors with flat locating edges. Their wide diameter makes it easier to direct the production of semen into the graduated test-tubes to which they are attached. The plastic is non-toxic and the funnel and test-tube arrangement is held in position on a stainless steel stand. Some patients find it difficult to produce a specimen by masturbation. To alleviate this problem sperm can be produced through intercourse using a seminal collection condom (Rocket Medical, Watford, UK) (Figure 11.3). These are

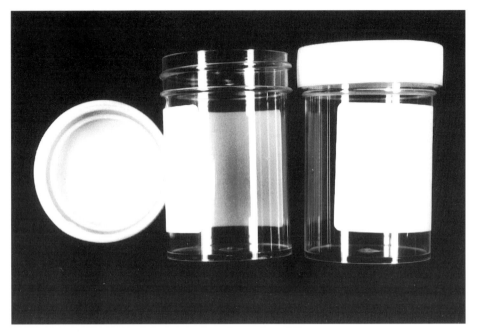

Figure 11.2. Specimen jars used for semen collection at NURTURE, supplied by LIP Equipment and Services Ltd, Shipley, UK.

manufactured from inert silicone rubber, are non-spermicidal and contain a patient identification label on the transport bag.

Chemicals used for in-house production of cryoprotectant media are available from Sigma UK Ltd (Poole, UK). Plastic disposables and glassware can be obtained from Scientific Laboratory Supplies Ltd (Nottingham, UK).

### *Packaging*

Semen is frozen in ampoules held on canes (Planer Products Ltd, Sunbury, UK) or straws stored in visitubes (Rocket Medical, Watford, UK). The ampoules, usually 1.5 ml in volume, are available with different coloured top inserts. Rocket Medical provide a complete range of materials for cryopreserving sperm in straws (Figure 11.3). Polyvinyl chloride straws are available in ten standard colours: clear, black, brown, red, green, blue, purple, yellow and pink; two sizes: 0.25 and 0.5 ml; and are 13 cm long. A further ten different colours are also available to special order: dark green, bright red, turquoise, orange, light blue, salmon, wine red, putty coloured, pale yellow and pistacchio green. One end of these straws is factory sealed. Polyvinyl alcohol (PVA) powder which solidifies when wet is used for sealing the open end of the straw. This is

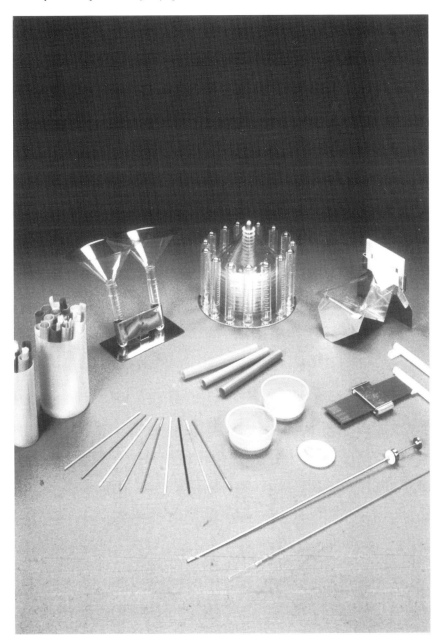

Figure 11.3. Items commonly used for the cryopreservation of human semen. Photograph by kind permission of Rocket Medical, Watford, UK.

available in 0.5 kg bags and in eight colours: white, black, red, green, blue, purple, yellow and orange. Non-smudge marker pens suitable for labelling samples stored in liquid nitrogen are also available from Rocket Medical.

The straws are held together between a metal clip with a plastic lining, and a multiple suction head connects to the top of the straws (Figure 11.3). This unit is connected by tubing to any laboratory vacuum pump providing a negative pressure. Also available from Rocket Medical (Figure 11.3) are plastic reservoirs to hold the diluted semen during the filling procedure. These reservoirs are clinically clean and for single use. A stainless steel stand is available to hold the reservoir, and a comb and guide fitment is available for creating air pockets in the open end of the straw after filling prior to the addition of the sealing powder. The filled and sealed straws are held in visitubes, which are available in ten colours, and are stored in clear plastic goblets (Figure 11.3).

## *Cryopreservation equipment*

### *Vapour freezing*

Those practitioners who decide to cryopreserve spermatozoa in the non-circulating vapour phase of liquid nitrogen need only purchase the vessels required for storage (Figure 11.4). The visitubes containing the straws are simply held in position in the vapour by holding with forceps, usually wedged in place with the vessel lid.

### *Programmable freezing*

The Kryo 10 (Planer Products Ltd, Sunbury, UK) (Figure 11.5) is a compact benchtop-controlled rate freezer operating in the range, 30 °C to −180 °C. The Kryo 10 allows both vertical and horizontal controlled rate freezing. An alternative to the Kryo 10 is the Kryosave freezer. This is the latest in the Planer range and is designed specifically as a low cost freezer for laboratories routinely freezing similar samples using an established single protocol, but also allows the practitioner to store individual programmes. The Freeze Control CL863 (CryoLogic Pty Ltd, Mt Waverley, Australia) (Figure 11.6) is a small, controlled rate freezer operating in the range, 40 to −86 °C. It operates on less than one litre of liquid nitrogen per hour and has no requirement for pressurised vessels or pumps. Hence, it is portable, economical and quiet, making it ideal for transport in vitro fertilisation (IVF) and fieldwork, where it can be run from a custom power pack.

Principles and practice of cryopreservation

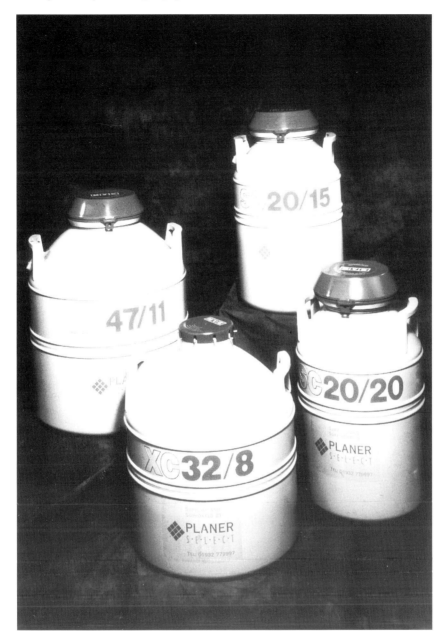

Figure 11.4. Vessels commonly used for the storage of cryopreserved human semen. Photograph by kind permission of Planer Products Ltd, Sunbury, UK.

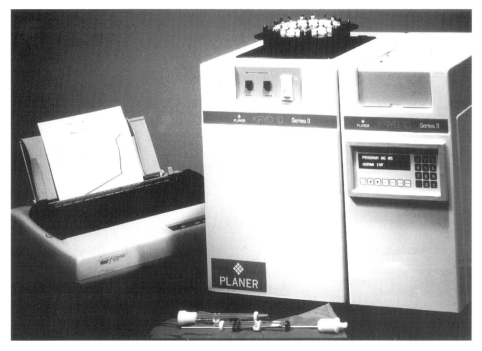

Figure 11.5. Kryo 10 series programmable freezer. Photograph by kind permission of Planer Products Ltd, Sunbury, UK.

### *Storage vessels*

Jencons Scientific Ltd, (Leighton Buzzard, UK) is the exclusive distributor for Taylor Wharton cryogenic refrigerators and containers (Figure 11.4) and accessories, including cryogloves, protective aprons, transfer and filling hoses for liquid nitrogen, protective glasses, dipping sticks, measuring rods, etc. Liquid nitrogen is available from BOC Ltd (Guildford, UK).

### Semen collection

Semen samples for use in AI programmes or for analysis during fertility investigations are usually produced by masturbation and collected directly into a suitable sterile, non-toxic, screw-topped jar (Figure 11.2). Where sterility is of particular importance, the hands and penis should be washed before collection. In all cases it is desirable to collect the entire ejaculate and avoid accidental loss or spillage. The sample is then transported to the laboratory as quickly as possible with care being taken to avoid extremes of temperature, for example < 20 °C or > 36 °C. Commonly, ejaculates are maintained at room temperature. In cases of poor semen quality it is often desirable to collect the first sperm-rich

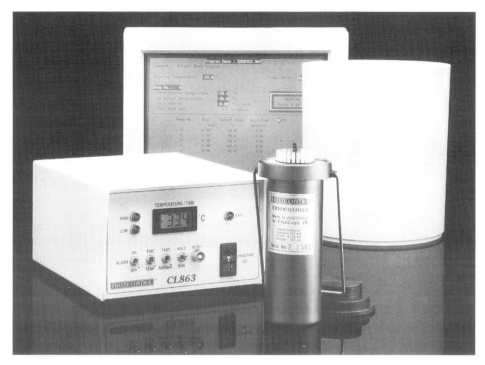

Figure 11.6. The FREEZE CONTROL CL863 User Programmable System. Photograph kindly supplied by Hunter Scientific Ltd, Widdington, UK; Distributor for Cryologic Pty Ltd, Mt Waverley, Australia.

fraction of the ejaculate separately from the remainder by directing the semen into two receptacles during ejaculation. For some men the production of a semen sample by masturbation is either not possible or unacceptable for a variety of reasons. *Coitus interruptus* is frequently used for sampling in these situations, but this may be unsatisfactory as it is difficult to ensure the collection of a complete, uncontaminated sample. The use of ordinary condoms is contraindicated for most applications due to their spermicidal qualities; however, the collection of a complete toxin-free ejaculate during coitus can be achieved by using non-spermicidal condoms made of silicone rubber (Rocket Medical, Watford, UK). Each condom is supplied with a clip for sealing the condom after the collection, a label for identification, and a sealable plastic bag for transporting the sample to the laboratory. Some religious codes or practices may require that a small pinhole is made in the condom before use, in which case it may be desirable to transfer the sample to a separate container immediately after collection.

**Washing procedure for glassware**

Where possible, it is beneficial to use disposable plasticware (Scientific Laboratory Supplies Ltd, Nottingham, UK). If the use of glassware for the preparation of cyroprotective media is unavoidable, the following protocol should be used in the cleaning process.

1. The glassware should be rinsed and sonicated in a recognised tissue culture cleaning agent such as Sebonex (ICN Biomedicals Ltd, Thame, UK) or a biological cleaning agent (Sigma UK Ltd, Poole, UK). Sonication is usually performed for about 30 minutes followed by extensive rinsing of the glassware in distilled water to remove all traces of the cleaning agents.
2. The glassware is then covered in aluminium foil or placed in an autoclave bag and labelled with autoclave tape. The glassware is heat-sterilised for approximately 2 hours at about 180 °C, until the autoclave tape shows that the sterilisation has been completed.

**Cryoprotective diluents**

There are two designs of diluent media in use today. Those based on an egg yolk-citrate medium with glycerol as the sole cryoprotective agent, and a modified Tyrode's medium containing three cryoprotectants: glycerol, glycine and sucrose. The latter formulation was developed by Mahadevan and Trounson in 1983 and does not require the addition of egg yolk, and it is this feature which makes it a favoured cryoprotection diluent for the preservation of surgically collected spermatozoa at NURTURE.

*Egg yolk formulations*

*Formulation 1. Matheson–Carlborg–Gemzell medium (1969)*

1. 20 ml yolk is separated from chicken eggs and heat-treated at 56 °C for 30 minutes.
2. Stock solutions of 3% trisodium citrate and 5.5% glucose are prepared using distilled water.
3. 39 ml 3% trisodium citrate, 26 ml 5.5% glucose and 15 ml glycerol are mixed together.
4. 1.5 g glycine and 0.1 g erythromycin are added to this mixture. This solution is now filtered through a 0.22 µm filter (Millipore UK Ltd, Watford, UK or Gelman Sciences Ltd, Northampton, UK) in order to sterilise it.
5. 20 ml heat-treated egg yolk is now added to this solution. The pH can be adjusted to 7.3 using 1.4% sodium bicarbonate solution.

*Principles and practice of cryopreservation*

6. The mixture is freeze-stored in 30 ml aliquots at −20 °C.

*Formulation 2*

1. 10 ml separated egg yolk is heat-treated at 56 °C for 30 minutes.
2. 2 g trisodium citrate, 1.6 g sucrose, 0.2 g glycine and 0.1 g erythromycin are made up to a volume of 78.9 ml in distilled water.
3. 21.3 ml glycerol is added to this solution, mixed and subsequently filtered through a 0.22 µm filter for sterilisation. To each 30 ml volume of glycerol-citrate buffer, 30 ml egg yolk is added and the mixture is freeze-stored at −20 °C.

Egg yolk-citrate media has been used for the cryopreservation of human sperm for many years. With the need to cryopreserve very poor sperm, such as epididymal sperm recovered for new microinjection procedures in assisted conception units, the egg yolk formulation is not an appropriate medium, largely because of the amount of extraneous material that results from using egg yolk. A cryoprotective diluent which is an alternative to egg yolk-citrate for sperm freezing, but is more suitable for these specimens, is the modified Tyrode's medium developed by Mahadevan and Trounson in 1983, which they called human sperm preservation medium (HSPM). A formulation based on HSPM is used at NURTURE (Table 11.1). An alternative, Sperm Freeze (Microm UK Ltd, Thame, UK), is a HEPES buffered cryopreservation medium based on glycerol.

## Dilution of semen samples with cryoprotectant diluent

Upon arrival at the laboratory, semen samples can be placed in an incubator at about 36 °C for liquefaction to occur, or preferentially kept at room temperature on the laboratory bench. Liquefaction usually takes between 10 and 30 minutes depending on the sample, and as soon as it is complete semen is mixed well and a small amount is removed for microscopic examination. Samples used for an AI programme would normally be expected to have a sperm concentration in excess of 50 million spermatozoa per ml with more than 50% showing good forward motility. The cryoprotectant diluent is commonly added to an ejaculate at room temperature. To avoid the damaging effects due to volume changes in the spermatozoon as a result of a response to the cryoprotectant itself, the cryoprotectant is added slowly in drop-wise fashion with continual swirling of the ejaculate mixture. An equal volume of cryoprotectant is added to the ejaculate (1:1), ratio the final concentration of glycerol in the diluted semen being about 8% in these formulations. Once the cryoprotectant has been added to the semen, the sample is left at room temperature for a minimum period of 10 minutes to allow the cryoprotectant to enter the cell and

Table 11.1. *Diluent formulation used at NURTURE for the cryopreservation of human spermatozoa*

| Chemical | Weight (g) |
| --- | --- |
| Sodium chloride | 2.900 |
| Potassium chloride | 0.200 |
| Sodium lactate syrup | 0.379 |
| Magnesium sulphate | 0.060 |
| Sodium hydrogen phosphate.$2H_2O$ | 0.025 |
| Sodium bicarbonate | 1.300 |
| HEPES | 2.380 |
| Sucrose | 8.590 |
| Glycine | 5.000 |
| Erythromycin | 0.025 |
| Human serum albumin | 2.000 |

*Notes:*
These chemicals should be completely dissolved before adding 75 ml of glycerol. Make up to 500 ml with distilled water. This solution is then filtered through a 0.22 μm filter to sterilise.

for the spermatozoon to complete the volume changes that it will be undergoing during this phase.

**Cryopreservation of very poor semen samples**

Techniques for the treatment of male infertility such as intracytoplasmic sperm injection (ICSI), which requires only a single viable spermatozoon to be manually delivered into an oocyte to achieve successful fertilisation, have changed our views about which sperm specimens should be cryopreserved. Even if there is no motility after thawing, the viability can be determined by incubating the recovered immotile sperm with hypo-osmotic medium. Viable spermatozoa will curl their tails when exposed to this medium and these spermatozoa can be subsequently used for ICSI. With this technical advance we are now required to freeze and thaw extremely poor samples for use in clinical treatment. The authors have found that successful cryopreservation and recovery of these specimens, rendering them suitable for microinjection, is achieved optimally in modified Tyrode's (HSPM) diluent and avoids the problems of debris associated with the egg yolk-citrate diluents. The methods described in the following section are used at NURTURE for the cryopreservation of these specimens.

### *Surgically recovered sperm*

Men who are azoospermic for a variety of reasons can be treated with assisted conception techniques by surgically aspirating sperm from the testes. To avoid the patient undergoing a second operation, sperm remaining after treatment can be frozen and thawed for subsequent assisted conception attempts. The spermatozoa are diluted in embryo culture medium to about 0.25 ml. HSPM-based diluent is added very slowly in drop-wise fashion until a 1:1 ratio is achieved. The resultant 0.5 ml of solution is aspirated into two 0.25 ml straws and prepared for freezing.

### *Preparation of very poor ejaculates*

Ejaculates containing very few sperm, or severely asthenozoospermic sperm, can be cryopreserved and used for a number of subsequent assisted conception attempts. The ejaculate is collected as a split ejaculate, the first fraction collected separately from the remainder, and is allowed to liquefy. Depending on the sperm content, either the first part or both parts are layered over a 90% and 45% discontinuous PureSperm (Scandinavian IVF Science AB, Gothenburg, Sweden) gradient. These are centrifuged at 500 $g$ for 10 minutes after which the bottom 0.5 ml of the 90% fraction is removed with a sterile glass Pasteur pipette. This fraction is mixed with 1 ml of embryo culture medium. The mixture is centrifuged at 250 $g$ for 5 minutes. After the supernatant is carefully removed, the pellet is resuspended in 1 ml of embryo culture medium and centrifuged again at 250 $g$ for 5 minutes to remove traces of PureSperm. The final sperm pellet, in embryo culture medium, is made up to 0.25–0.5 ml. The cryoprotectant diluent is added very slowly in drop-wise fashion until a 1:1 ratio is achieved. The resultant mixture is left at room temperature for a minimum of 10 minutes prior to loading into 0.25 ml straws for freezing.

### Packaging the semen sample ready for cryopreservation

Semen cryopreservation diluent mixtures are commonly frozen in straws although some practitioners still prefer to freeze in ampoules.

### *Straws*

Plastic straws for semen cryopreservation are available in two sizes: 0.5 and 0.25 ml, and in a variety of colours. Each straw has a pair of cotton plugs at one end enclosing a small quantity of PVA powder which will gel on contact with liquids. This automatically forms an efficient seal to the top of the straw when it is filled. The open end of the straw can then be similarly sealed by pushing it into more PVA powder. Prior to filling, the straws may be labelled or marked for identification and they are then packed in plastic-lined stainless steel clips in batches of 20 for 0.25 ml straws, or 15 for 0.5 ml straws. The straws are all aligned with the plugged ends uppermost and semen is drawn up into them, either singularly or a clip at a time by locating a suction manifold over the upper ends. This suction head is connected by flexible tubing to any standard laboratory pump providing a steady vacuum of 300–600 mm of mercury. To accommodate expansion during freezing, a small air space is introduced into the column of semen before sealing the lower end. This is achieved by pushing the clip full of straws onto a plastic comb and then removing them swiftly. After filling, the straws are wiped to remove excess semen and the open ends are pushed firmly and evenly into coloured PVA powder to form a plug about 4–5 mm long. The powder may be held in a suitable shallow container or compressed firmly into a clean glass plate to a depth of about 5 mm. It is recommended that the powder be discarded after each batch to prevent contamination or inefficient sealing of subsequent batches. When the straws have been filled and sealed, they are removed from the clips and can then be wiped clean or washed in a water bath and dried. This removes powder and semen from the outside, which will help to prevent the straws sticking together during freezing.

### *Ampoules*

As an alternative to straws, semen can be loaded into 1.5 ml glass or plastic ampoules. To allow for expansion during the freezing process, a gap is left at the top of the ampoule before sealing. The ampoules are subsequently loaded into canes ready for freezing. Before the spermatozoa undergo the freezing process, a sperm assessment must be performed just prior to loading in order to determine any effect that the cryoprotectant diluent may have had.

## Cryopreservation techniques for human sperm

### *Cryopreserving sperm in non-circulating liquid nitrogen vapour*

The method of suspending the sperm-diluent mixture, whether contained in straws or ampoules, vertically in the non-circulating vapour phase of liquid nitrogen (Bunge *et al.* 1954) is the simplest way to freeze spermatozoa. Filled straws contained in visitubes, or ampoules held on canes, are suspended in the non-circulating vapour of liquid nitrogen. The most common way of doing this is to position long forceps which hold the visitubes or canes in the liquid nitrogen vapour by jamming them in the neck of the storage vessel using the lid. The straws are kept in the vapour for about half an hour whereby an estimated freezing rate of about $-10\,°C$ per minute down to a temperature of about $-80\,°C$ is obtained The straws are subsequently plunged into liquid nitrogen at $-196\,°C$.

### *Modifications of vapour freezing*

In 1991 Kobayashi *et al.* published their findings after cryopreserving human spermatozoa in cryosyringes held horizontally on a floating platform 3 cm above the surface of liquid nitrogen. In this report, a preliminary concentration of sperm from the entire ejaculate was prepared using Percoll density gradient centrifugation, and was diluted with cryopreservation medium, KS 11 (Kaneko *et al.* 1990). A freezing rate of $-37\,°C$ per minute was achieved with freezing completed within 5 minutes. They concluded that the quality of post-thaw recovery of spermatozoa was not compromised using this approach. They reported that this more rapid freeze is comparable to survival rates seen after conventional vertical vapour freezing and programmable freezing (Won 1989).

### *Programmable freezing of human semen*

Sperm can be frozen at a rate of $-1\,°C$ per minute from ambient temperature to $5\,°C$, followed by $-10\,°C$ per minute to $-85\,°C$. Once this temperature has been reached, the straws can be removed and plunged into liquid nitrogen for storage at $-196\,°C$. The Kryo 10 programmable freezer (Planer Products Ltd, Sunbury, UK) has the facility to freeze straws vertically or horizontally.

### *Dry ice pelletting*

Pelleting semen directly on dry ice, although used successfully in the past, is not in common usage today. Whichever method is preferred, the only true assessment of the success of the technique is the ability of the thawed sperm to fertilise an oocyte in vitro or the creation of a clinical pregnancy following insemination. Much work has been performed to determine the efficiency of these techniques.

## The effect of cryopreservation on the motility and fertility of spermatozoa

The general criteria used to indicate the viability of frozen-thawed spermatozoa has been the maintenance of motility, but of course this does not relate to a spermatozoon's fertilising capacity. The only true assessment of the success of a freezing technique is the ability of the thawed sperm to fertilise an oocyte in vitro, or the creation of a clinical pregnancy after direct insemination. Given that we have an appropriate cryoprotectant diluent and protocol for semen collection and dilution, the next step is to determine what effect, if any, these different freezing techniques have on the fertility of spermatozoa.

The ATP levels, percentage of sperm surviving the hypo-osmotic swelling test, survival time in vitro, ability to penetrate cervical mucus and the motility of sperm thawed after freezing are lower when compared with fresh sperm (Zhu et al. 1990). It was also observed by these authors that there was no significant difference between the percentage of zona-free hamster egg penetrations achieved by frozen-thawed sperm and fresh sperm, but the penetration index declined over time, indicating that fertility per se was not affected in human sperm as a result of the freeze-thaw process, but may be affected over an extended time in vitro. A time-dependent loss in motility resulting from sublethal cryodamage was shown by Alvarez and Storey in 1992. It had previously been shown (Hanson et al. 1982) that sperm survival in cervical mucus was significantly related to conception following insemination with fresh sperm. It is therefore feasible that any loss of motility due to a delayed process would markedly affect fecundity. One source of damage to sperm membranes resulting in a temperature- and time-dependent loss of motility was suggested to be that of lipid peroxidation due to the cryopreservation damage of the protective enzyme superoxide dismutase (Alvarez & Storey 1992). The freeze-thaw process would promote membrane lipid peroxidation such that the cell membranes lose their permeability barriers at a more rapid rate than would membranes from untreated cells, and thus shorten the lifetime of these cells. Another source of cryodamage which may have a time-dependent effect on spermatozoa is that of membrane stress in which the phase transitions encountered by the plasma membrane during the freeze-thaw make the membrane more prone to early fracture at the stress points (Alvarez & Storey 1993). There have been a number of studies to determine whether there is any significant difference in the effect on human spermatozoa of being frozen in the vapour phase of liquid nitrogen compared to the programmable method (Thachil & Jewett 1981; Taylor et al. 1982; Zhu et al. 1990). A number of these authors found no difference in the outcome of freezing from either method;

however McLaughlin *et al.* (1990) showed that the cooling rate within straws frozen in non-circulating liquid nitrogen vapour is very variable both between different positions in the straw and between replicate freezes. The shape of the cooling curves inside straws frozen by the programmable method, however, showed a similar shape thoughout the straw (McLaughlin *et al.* 1990). This difference in freezing uniformity between vapour and programmable freezing results in statistically less injury to the spermatozoa and a higher percentage of progressively motile sperm with a larger lateral head displacement after programmable freezing (McLaughlin *et al.* 1990). The vapour freezing technique however, is cheap and convenient, has been the standard method for the cryopreservation of human semen for many years, and is likley to remain so even though we now know that the method confers a statistically poorer freeze.

## The effect of thawing on the survival of cryopreserved spermatozoa

The optimal freezing rate of mammalian sperm is in the range, $-10\ ^\circ\text{C}$ per minute to $-100\ ^\circ\text{C}$ per minute (Polge 1980). Consequently, human sperm can be frozen and thawed successfully using a range of freezing and thawing procedures, as long as the freezing rate lies within this range and the thawing is rapid. Using motility as the criterion for a successful freeze-thaw, it has been demonstrated that a variety of thawing techniques will result in good recovery irrespective of the freezing method (Taylor *et al.* 1982). Most practitioners either rub the straw or the ampoule between their fingers or keep them at room temperature until they are thawed. Other methods of thawing for both the programmable freeze and vapour freeze techniques which have been tried are: (1) thawing at room temperature for 10 minutes followed by 37 °C for 10 minutes, (2) thawing in iced water for 10 minutes followed by 37 °C for 10 minutes, (3) thawing at 35 °C in a water bath for 12 seconds followed by 37 °C for 10 minutes, and (4) plunging the straws or ampoules into a 37 °C water bath directly until melted.

The actual technique of thawing does not appear to be critical, but the thaw must be rapid. It is important to avoid loss of sperm motility resulting from osmotic shock due to inappropriate preparation of the thawed sperm. Up to half of the recovered motile population can be lost if the contents of a 0.25 ml straw is mixed directly into 2 ml of culture media. At NURTURE we have found that the processing described in the following section results in minimal loss of spermatozoa caused by osmotic shock.

### *Removing sperm from the straws*

The straws are stored in liquid nitrogen at $-196\,^\circ\text{C}$. The appropriate number of straws are removed and thawed as previously described. The percentage recovery of motile cells will dictate the number of straws required for a particular procedure. Straws containing a motile population of around 20 million per millilitre would necessitate only two 0.25 ml straws to be thawed for direct insemination into the cervical canal, or possibly four straws or more if washing is used for direct intrauterine insemination. IVF procedures requiring frozen-thawed sperm would usually demand the thawing of two to four 0.25 ml straws depending on the number of oocytes to be inseminated.

For those procedures requiring the washing of frozen-thawed sperm from the cryoprotective medium into culture medium, the contents of the straws are first emptied over a 45 and 90% discontinuous PureSperm gradient as follows: a pair of scissors is flame-sterilised and the PVA plugged ends of the straws are cut. The open ends of the straws are placed over the PureSperm gradient. The factory plug can now be cut allowing the contents to trickle onto the PureSperm gradient. The semen-diluent mix is kept on the gradient for 5 minutes to allow equilibration at room temperature before the centrifugation and washing steps. Semen preparation is subsequently carried out in the same manner as for semen washing. This consists of a $500\,g$ centrifugation for 10 minutes, followed by two washing centrifugation steps, each of $250\,g$ for 5 minutes, until the sperm is recovered into culture media. The removal of the sample from ampoules is simply by aspirating with a pipette and the subsequent processing is the same as for sperm recovered from straws.

### *Simultaneous assessment of sperm motility and viability following cryopreservation*

A recently developed sperm viability kit, LIVE/DEAD *Ferti*light (Cambridge BioScience, Cambridge, UK), has been reported to be useful in assessing the quality of cryopreserved bovine spermatozoa in a time-dependent manner (Garner *et al.* 1994). It relies upon the incubation of spermatozoa within medium containing the nucleic acid stains propidium iodide and SYBR-14 (Cambridge BioScience, Cambridge, UK), living cell membranes being impermeable to the former but permeable to the latter. These dyes label cells more rapidly than conventional stains and may be excited with visible as well as with ultraviolet light, and living spermatozoa stained with SYBR-14 may be tracked, thereby facilitating rapid analysis of their motility and abundance. Hence, cell death can be monitored through a relatively rapid transition in staining from green (SYBR-14) to red (propidium iodide). We have modified this technique to assess the motility and viability of human spermatozoa, employing the following protocol.

1. The semen sample is prepared by 45 and 90% discontinuous Percoll (Pharmacia LKB Biotechnology, Uppsala, Sweden) gradient centrifugation, then diluted in 1 ml embryo culture medium.
2. SYBR-14 and propidium iodide are added to the 1 ml sample of diluted semen to a final concentration of 100 nM and 12 M, respectively.
3. The stained sample may be analysed following a 5–10 minute incubation.

*Storage*

The most convenient method of freezing human sperm with regards to their subsequent storage is to use straws. These can be packed in visitubes and placed in cannisters within liquid nitrogen refrigerators. The many different colours available for straws, sealing powder, visitubes and goblets, makes it possible to code each ejaculate in a variety of ways for systematic storage and retrieval, and for positive identification of the sample later on.

### Summary

Cryopreservation of human spermatozoa involves complex interactions between the cell membranes and the cryoprotectant diluent employed, which are temperature-dependent. Hence, there are a variety of methods available, each being more suitable for specific circumstances. Nevertheless, it is clear that precise control of rates of cooling and thawing is essential for the successful recovery of motile, viable cells. In this respect, appropriate analysis should be applied, the only physiologically meaningful end-points being fertilisation and pregnancy.

### References

Aloia R. C., Curtin C. C. & Gordon L. M. (1988) *Lipid Domains and the Relationship to Membrane Function*. Alan R. Liss, New York.

Alvarez J. G. & Storey B. T. (1992) Evidence for increased lipid peroxidative damage and loss of superoxide dismutase activity as a mode of sublethal cryodamage to human sperm during cryopreservation. *Journal of Andrology* **13**, 232–241.

Alvarez J. G. & Storey B. T. (1993) Evidence that membrane stress contributes more than lipid peroxidation to sublethal cryodamage in cryopreserved human sperm : glycerol and other polyols as sole cryoprotectant. *Journal of Andrology* **14**, 199–209.

Bedford J. M. & Calvin H. I. (1974) The occurrence and possible functional significance of s-s crosslinks in sperm heads, with particular reference to eutherian mammals. *Journal of Experimental Zoology* **188**, 137–156.

Blackshaw A. W. (1954) The prevention of temperature shock of bull and ram semen. *Australian Journal of Biological Sciences* **7,** 573–582.

Boggs J. M. & Rangaraj G. (1985) Phase transitions and fatty acid spin label behaviour in interdigitated lipid phases induced by glycerol and polymyxin. *Biochimica et Biophysica Acta* **816,** 221–233.

Bredderman P. J. & Foote R. H. (1969) Volume of stressed bull spermatozoa and protoplast droplets, and the relationshp of cell size to motility and fertility. *Journal of Dairy Science* **28,** 496–501.

Bunge R. G., Keettel W. & Sherman J. (1954) Clinical use of frozen sperm, report of four cases. *Fertility and Sterility* **5,** 520–529.

Carruthers A. & Melchior D. L. (1988a) Effects of lipid environment on membrane transport. The human erythrocyte sugar transport protein/lipid bilayer system. *Annual Review of Physiology* **50,** 257–271.

Carruthers A. & Melchior D. L. (1988b) Role of bilayer lipids in governing membrane transport processes. In: *Lipid Domains and the Relationship to Membrane Function.* (R. C. Aloia, C. C. Curtin, L. M. Gordon, eds), Alan R. Liss, New York, pp. 201–225.

Chang M. C. & Walton A. (1940) The effects of low temperature and acclimatisation on the respiratory activity and survival of ram spermatozoa. *Proceedings of the Royal Society of London, Series B* **129,** 517–527.

Darin-Bennett A., Poulos A. & White I. G. (1974) The phospholipid and phospholipid-bound fatty acids and aldehydes of dog and fowl spermatozoa. *Journal of Reproduction and Fertility* **41,** 471–474.

Darin-Bennett A. & White I. G. (1977) Influence of the cholesterol content of mammalian spermatozoa on susceptibility to cold shock. *Cryobiology* **14,** 466–470.

Darin-Bennett A., White I. G. & Hoskins D. D. (1977) Phospholipids and phospholipid-bound fatty acids and aldehydes of spermatozoa and seminal plasma of rhesus monkeys. *Journal of Reproduction and Fertility* **49,** 119–122.

De Gier J. (1989) Osmotic properties of liposomes. In: *Water Transport in Biological Membranes. Vol 1. From Model Membranes to Isolated Cells.* (G. Benga, ed.), CRC Press, Boca Raton, pp. 77–98.

De Leeuw F. E., Colenbrander B. & Verklerj A. J. (1988) Cold-induced changes in bovine sperm plasma membrane: a freeze-fracture study. *XI International Congress on Animal Reproduction and Artificial Insemination (Dublin)* 3, No. 237.

Drevius L. -O. & Erickson H. (1966) Osmotic swelling of mammalian spermatozoa. *Experimental Cell Research* **42,** 136–156.

Duncan A.E. (1988) *Studies of the effects of freezing rate on the cryosurvival of ram spermatozoa.* PhD Thesis. University of London.

Eddy E.M. (1988) The Spermatozoon. In: *The Physiology of Reproduction.* (E. Knobil, J. Neil, eds). Raven Press, New York, pp. 27–68.

Fiser P. S. & Fairfull R. W. (1989) The effect of glycerol-related osmotic changes on post thaw motility and acrosomal integrity of ram spermatozoa. *Cryobiology* **26,** 64–69.

Garner D. L., Johnson L. A., Yue S. T., Roth B. L. & Haugland R. P. (1994) Dual DNA staining assessment of bovine sperm viability using SYBR-14 and propidium iodide. *Journal of Andrology* **15,** 620–629.

Hammerstedt R. H., Graham J. K. & Nolan J. P. (1990) Cryopreservation of mammalian sperm: what we ask them to survive. *Journal of Andrology* **11,** 73–87.

Hammerstedt R. H., Keith A. D., Snipes W. C., Amann R. P., Arruda D. & Griel L. C. Jr. (1978) Use of spin labels to evaluate effects of cold shock and osmolality on sperm. *Biology of Reproduction* **18**, 686–696.

Hammerstedt R. H. & Parks J. E. (1987) Changes in sperm surfaces associated with epididymal transit. *Journal of Reproduction and Fertility* (supplement) **34**, 133–149.

Hanson F. W., Overstreet J. W. & Katz D. F. (1982) A study of the relationship of motile sperm numbers in cervical mucus 48 hours after artificial insemination with subsequent fertility. *American Journal of Obstetrics and Gynecology* **143**, 85–90.

Heape W. (1897) The artificial insemination of mammals and subsequent possible fertilisation or impregnation of their ova. *Proceedings of the Royal Society of London* **61**, 52–63.

Hoagland H. & Pincus G. (1942) Revival of mammalian sperm after immersion in liquid nitrogen. *Journal of General Physiology* **25**, 337–344.

Hochachka P. W. (1986) Defence strategies against hypoxia and hypothermia. *Science* **231**, 234–241.

Hochachka P. W. & Guppy M. (1987) *Metabolic Arrest and the Control of Biological Time*. Harvard University Press, Cambridge.

Holt W. V. & North R. D. (1984) Partially irreversible cold-induced lipid phase transitions in mammalian sperm plasma membrane domains: freeze-fracture study. *Journal of Experimental Zoology* 230, 473–483.

Inskeep P. B. & Hammerstedt R. H. (1985) Endogenous metabolism by sperm in response to altered cellular ATP requirements. *Journal of Cellular Physiology* **123**, 180–190.

Jacobi L. (1765) *Kunstliche Fischzucht*. Hannover, Magazin.

Jeyendran R. S., Van der Ven H. H., Perez-Pelaez M., Crabo B. G. & Zaneveld L. J. D. (1984) Development of an assay to assess the functional integrity of the human sperm membrane and its relationship to other semen characteristics. *Journal of Reproduction and Fertility* **70**, 219–228.

Kaneko S., Lee H. K., Kobayashi T., Oda T., Ohno T. & Iizuka R. (1990) Cryopreservation of washed and concentrated human sperm and its application to AIH. *Journal of Fertilization and Implantation (Tokyo)* **7**, 120–123.

Kobayashi T., Kaneko S., Hara I., Park J. Y., Aoki R., Ohno T. & Nozawa S. (1991) A simplified technique for freezing human sperm for AIH: cryosyringe/floating platform of liquid nitrogen vapour. *Archives of Andrology* **27**, 55–60.

Luyet B. J. & Hodapp E. L. (1938) Revival of frog's spermatozoa vitrified in liquid air. *Proceedings of the Society of Experimental Biology and Medicine* **39**, 433–434.

McLaughlin E. A., Ford W. C. L. & Hull M. G. R. (1990) A comparison of the freezing of human semen in the uncirculated vapour above liquid nitrogen and in a commercial semi-programmable freezer. *Human Reproduction* **5**, 724–728.

Mahadevan M. & Trounson A. (1983) Effect of cryoprotective media and dilution methods on the preservation of human spermatozoa. *Andrologia* **15**, 355.

Mantegazza P. (1866) Sullo sperma umano. *Rendiconti dell'Istituto Lombardo di Scienze e Lettere* **3**, 183–196.

Matheson G. W., Carlborg L. & Gemzell C. (1969) Frozen human semen for artificial insemination. *American Journal of Obstetrics and Gynecology* **104**, 495–501.

Mazur P. (1984) Freezing of living cells: mechanisms and implications. *American Journal of Physiology* **247**, 125–142.

Mazur P., Leibo S. P. & Miller R. H. (1974) Permeability of the bovine red cell to glycerol in hyperosmotic solutions at various temperatures. *The Journal of Membrane Biology* **15**, 107–136.

Mazur P. & Miller R. H. (1976) Permeability of the human erythrocyte to glycerol in 1 and 2 M solutions at 0 or 20 °C. *Cryobiology* **13**, 507–522.

Mazur P. & Rajotte R. V. (1981) Permeability of the 17 day fetal rat pancreas to glycerol and dimethylsulfoxide. *Cryobiology* **18**, 1–16.

Milovanov V. K. (1934) *Iskustvennoe osemenenie, S.L . zivotnyh* (artificial insemination of livestock). Seljhozgiz, Moscow.

O'Leary T. S. & Levin I. W. (1984) Ramen spectroscopic study of an interdigitated lipid bilayer dipalmitoylphosphatidylcholine dispersed in glycerol. *Biochimica et Biophysica Acta* **776**, 185–189.

Phillips P. H. (1939) Preservation of bull semen. *Journal of Biological Chemistry* **130**, 415.

Polge C. (1980) Freezing of spermatozoa. In: *Low Temperature Preservation in Medicine and Biology*. (M. S. Ashwood-Smith, J. Ferrant, eds) Pitman, Bath, pp. 45–53.

Polge C., Smith A. V. & Parkes A. S. (1949) Revival of spermatozoa after vitrification and dehydration at low temperatures. *Nature* **164**, 666.

Poulos A., Darin-Bennett A. & White I. G. (1973) The phospholipid-bound fatty acids and aldehydes of mammalian spermatozoa. *Comparative Biochemistry and Physiology, Series B* **46B**, 541–549.

Quinn P. J. (1989) Principles of membrane stability and phase behaviour under extreme conditions. *Journal of Bioenergetics and Biomembranes* **21**, 3–19.

Quinn P. J., Chow P. Y. W. & White I. G. (1980) Evidence that phospholipid protects ram spermatozoa from cold shock at a plasma membrane site. *Journal of Reproduction and Fertility* **60**, 403–407.

Rudenko S. V., Gapochenko S. D. & Bondarenko U. A. (1984) Effect of glycerol on the capacitance and conductivity of bilayer lipid membranes. *Biophysics* **29**, 245–249.

Schneider U. (1986) Cryobiological principles of embryo freezing. *Journal of In Vitro Fertilization and Embryo Transfer* **3**, 3–9.

Shaffner C. S., Henderson E. W. & Card C. G. (1941) Viability of spermatozoa of the chicken under various environmental conditions. *Poultry Science* **20**, 259–265.

Singer S. J. & Nicolson G. L. (1972) The fluid mosaic model of the structure of cell membranes. *Science* **175**, 720–731.

Spallanzani L. (1776) Opuscoli di Fisica Animale e Vegetabile Opuscola 2. Observationi e sperienze intorno ai vermicelli spermatici dell'homo e degli animali. Modena.

Steponkus P. L. & Lynch D. V. (1989) Freeze\thaw induced destabilization of the plasma membrane and the effects on cold acclimations. *Journal of Bioenergetics and Biomembranes* **21**, 21–41.

Thachil J. V. & Jewett M. A. S. (1981) Preservation techniques for human semen. *Fertility and Sterility* **35**, 546–548.

Taylor P. J., Wilson J., Haycock R. & Weger J. (1982) A comparison of freezing and thawing methods for the cryopreservation of human semen. *Fertility and Sterility* **37**, 100–103.

Van Leeuwenhoek A. (1677) Observationes de Anthonu Lewenhoeck, de Natis e Semine Genitali Animaculis. *Philosophical Transactions of the Royal Society of London* **12**, 1040–1043.

Watson P. F. (1976) The protection of ram and bull spermatozoa by the low density fraction of egg yolk during storage at 5 °C and deep-freezing. *Journal of Thermal Biology* **1,** 137–141.

Watson P. F. (1979) The preservation of semen in mammals. In: *Oxford Reviews of Reproductive Biology, vol. 1.* (C. A. Finn, ed.), Oxford University Press, Oxford, p. 283.

Watson P. F. (1981a) The effects of cold shock on sperm cell membranes. In: *Effects of Low Temperatures on Biological Membranes*. (G. J. Morris, A. Clarke, eds), Academic Press, London, pp. 189–218.

Watson P. F. (1981b) The roles of lipid and protein in the protection of ram spermatozoa at 5 °C by egg-yolk lipoprotein. *Journal of Reproduction and Fertility* **62,** 483–492.

Watson P. F. & Morris G. J. (1987) Cold shock injury in animal cells. In: *Temperature and Animal Cells.* (K. Bowler, B. J. Fuller, eds), Society of Experimental Biology Symposium No. 41. The Company of Biologists, Cambridge. pp. 311–340.

Won W. K. (1989) Studies on the cryopreservation of concentrated human sperm, and its application to AID. *Keio Journal of Medicine* **66,** 679–688.

Zhu W.-J., Liu X.-G., Li S.-Q., Wen R.-Q. & Wang C.-X. (1990) Human sperm cryobiological characteristics: comparative cryopreservation techniques. *Archives of Andrology* **24,** 95–96.

# 12
## Donor sperm banking

JOAN P. CRICH

### Introduction

Cryobanking of semen was a logical sequel to the development of cryopreservation. Initial applications were mainly in the animal industry but since the 1970's human sperm banks have become established in many parts of the world. The need for quarantine of donor semen for at least 6 months, in order to retest donors for the human immunodeficiency virus (HIV) and other infections, is the main impetus for the present day popularity of semen banking. There are other indications for long-term storage of semen. Prior to treatment that may compromise a man's future fertility, such as chemotherapy for malignant disease and surgical removal of testicular tumours, a patient may have his semen cryopreserved especially if he has not had children or completed his family. Some men may elect to have their semen frozen prior to vasectomy but this does not seem to have become a popular indication. Theoretically at least, several samples from an oligozoospermic patient could be stored as they are produced and later on pooled for use during artificial insemination or other assisted conception treatments. Men who have problems masturbating on demand such as on the day of an assisted conception procedure, may come in at their convenience and do so in advance of the treatment. The same also applies to men who will be absent at the time of their wives' treatment or normal fertile couples whose husbands have to be away for long periods.

The bulk of semen stored at any point in time in most semen banks, however, comprise donor samples. There are a number of indications for use of donor semen such as severe oligo-, astheno- and/or teratozoospermia, azoospermia, the presence of seminal antisperm antibodies and the risk of transmission of genetic disease from the male parent to a male offspring. These are however relative indications because recent developments in male infertility treatment such as epididymal sperm recovery and intracytoplasmic sperm injection have provided a large number of men with the opportunity for genetic parenthood. Pre-implantation genetic diagnosis and transfer of embryos not carrying the disorder, is now providing similar opportunities for affected men and it is obvious that the number of disorders that can be screened for in this way will increase in the future. Donor insemination will however continue to be required for many patients.

Much is still unknown about optimal freezing and thawing methods and this has given rise to a plethora of techniques. Most authorities in this area of scientific endeavour agree that provided a method achieves consistently good results in relation to pregnancy rates in the recipients, the centre should continue with that method rather than trying to change to an unfamiliar technique. This writer was involved in setting up and running the first donor sperm bank under the National Health Service scheme of the UK. The following account is based on experience gained from the successful operation of this unit for the past 21 years.

### Recruitment of donors

Donors may be recruited in many ways, using the media or internally, depending on the size of the establishment requiring them. In a town where there is a university, notices may be put up on the campus notice boards. When a medical school is in the vicinity, lecturers, when approached, will mention a fertility clinic's need for donors to students during lectures. There are also many other places to advertise such as surgery waiting rooms or public rooms, as in a library. The wording needs to be just enough to explain the situation, without being explicit. To state that there is a fertility clinic close by, which is in need of sperm donors, and give a telephone number from which further information may be obtained, is usually enough. Full confidentiality must be assured, and of course mention is made that expenses will be paid. Once a few donors have been recruited, others follow; word seems to get around. There is presently a trend to recruit from amongst men who have already fathered children of their own. This will overcome problems with student donors who are of unproven fertility and tend to change sexual partners more frequently, with the result that sexually transmitted diseases are more likely in this class of donors. Fertile sperm donors can be recruited from vasectomy clinics, antenatal clinics and through the press.

### Counselling of donors

The initial counselling of a donor is of the utmost importance. One cannot stress too strongly the integrity and commitment required from a donor, but more than this he must be made aware of emotions that as yet, he has never experienced. He has to understand the fact that should insemination with his sperm be successful, somewhere there will be a child born that he will never know, have no connection with whatsoever, but will nevertheless be the child's biological father. It is really difficult to project or suppose what ones feelings could be in this situation but this is what donors are asked to do. If he is a successful donor, there could be ten such children, which is the maximum allowed for each donor in the UK by the Human Fertilisation and Embryology Authority (HFEA). This may be stating the obvious but deliberate attempts have to be made to ensure that the donors' own joy in parenthood is in no way diminished, because of their willingness at this time to help infertile couples achieve a family. External counselling by an independent counsellor must be offered to all donors. This is especially important because some who come forward initially to become donors may be rejected later on as a result of subnormal sperm parameters or a positive screening test for disease. All prospective donors should be prepared psychologically for such eventuality and adequate backup support and medical care made available.

### Screening and selection of donors

Key activities during screening and selection of donors can be divided into history taking, analysis of a semen sample and clinical examination and laboratory tests, although opinions vary as to their correct sequence. The aim is to carry out the easiest and less costly activities first before going on to the more invasive and costly tests for those donors who successfully negotiate the first stage of the process. Screening of donors is aimed at prevention of disease transmission to either or both the recipient mother and offspring, and selection of only those who have seminal parameters most likely to achieve pregnancy in the recipient. Screening starts with a complete medical and family history. They are asked whether they have had urethral discharge, genital warts or ulcers or herpes infection at anytime in the past. Historical markers for HIV are sought for such as homosexuality, intravenous drug abuse, receipt of pooled plasma products such as Factor 8 before the era of heat treatment of these products, visit to areas with high prevalence of acquired immune deficiency syndrome and having sex with the inhabitants of those areas. Donors who have been sexual partners of any female belonging to any of these groups of individuals are also excluded. A donor is also not acceptable if there is a history of genetically inherited disorders anywhere in the family. The list of such disorders is opened ended and Table 12.1 shows the recommendations of the British Andrology Society (Barratt *et al.* 1993).

Table 12.1. *British Andrology Society recommended minimal genetic screening for gamete donors*

---

*The donor*

1. Familial disease with a major genetic component:

| | |
|---|---|
| Cleft lip | Congenital heart malformation |
| Cleft palate | Hypospadias |
| Clubfoot | Spina bifida |
| Congenital hip dislocation | |

2. Non-trivial Mendelian disorder:

| | |
|---|---|
| Albinism (general or ocular) | Hereditary hypercholesterolaemia |
| Haemoglobin disorder | Neurofibromatosis |
| Haemophilia | Tuberous sclerosis |

3. Familial disease with known or reliably indicated major genetic component:

| | |
|---|---|
| Asthma | Rheumatoid arthritis |
| Epileptic disorder | Severe hypertension |
| Juvenile diabetes mellitus | Severe refractive disorder |
| Psychosis | |

4. Detectable heterozygosity for ethnically prevalent autosomal recessive gene disorder

| | |
|---|---|
| β-thalassaemia | Cystic fibrosis (screening is optional) |
| Sickle-cell disease | Tay–Sachs disease |
| Glucose-6-phosphate dehydrogenase deficiency | |

5. Carrier of chromosomal rearrangement that may result in unbalanced gametes

*History of disorder in donor's parents or siblings*

1. Familial disease with a major genetic component (as above)

2. Non-trivial disorders showing Mendelian inheritance:
(a) Autosomal dominant or X-linked with donor not yet reached the age of onset (Huntington's disease).
(b) Autosomal dominant disorder with reduced penetrance (Marfan syndrome and Alport's disease)
(c) Autosomal recessive disorder which is common in the population (cystic fibrosis)

3. Chromosomal abnormality except if the donor has a normal karyotype.

---

*Source:* Adapted from Barratt *et al.* (1993)

A complete physical examination is carried out and this includes examination of the genital area. Tests are carried out on blood, urethral swabs and urine to exclude or detect sexually transmitted diseases or any other infection. Specific pathogens screened for include HIV, Hepatitis B and C viruses, *Chlamydia trachomatis*, cytomegalovirus (CMV), *Neisseria gonorrhoeae*,

*Ureaplasma urealyticum, Mycoplasma hominis, Trichomonas vaginalis, Treponema pallidum*. CMV requires special mention. A donor who is positive for CMV does not necessarily have to be rejected; however only women who are also positive for CMV should be inseminated with semen from such donors if these women agree. Seronegative recipients should only be inseminated with semen from CMV negative donors. All donors must have their ABO and Rhesus blood groups determined.

Semen must be produced on site at the first and subsequent visits. This is in order to ensure that it arrives fresh at the laboratory and to prevent substitute samples from people other than the donor. Obviously the semen sample from the donor must be of 'better than normal' quality to ensure survival of an acceptable number of spermatozoa after thawing. The standard which we require at our bank comprises of a volume of 1–5 ml, concentration of 60 million or more spermatozoa per millilitre of semen and a motility of 60% or more with very good progressive movement. Other parameters are according to the World Health Organization's criteria (WHO 1992) (see Chapter 8). There should be no increase in cellular content; this should be watched for in any sample produced by the same donor. If white blood cells are increased in number, microbiological investigations should be carried out and the responsible pathogen eradicated with antibiotics. There should also be no signs of anti-sperm antibody activity. It is of utmost importance that there is no increase in abnormal forms. The sperms should have a good post-thaw recovery and this should be checked for each time a batch of semen form a donor is frozen as this can vary in different samples produced by the same donor.

Prospective donors should be provided with relevant information sheets and guidelines so that they understand fully the legal as well as the moral obligations of becoming a sperm donor. In the UK, all donors must be registered by name and the code number allocated to them by the sperm bank, with the HFEA within 2 weeks of first using their semen samples for insemination. The Royal College of Obstetricians and Gynaecologists have produced an information leaflet for donors which briefly describes the need for donor semen, what makes an individual suitable to become a semen donor, the tests required before semen donation and those who are ineligible for donation based on their above average risk of contracting the HIV by reason of their lifestyle or treatment with Factor 8. The last page of the leaflet has a declaration to be signed by the donor before a clinician declaring that he had read the leaflet and understood that the high risk groups described in the leaflet should not donate semen, and that he understood the significance of the tests described. The clinician also signs in front of the donor declaring that he made sure the donor read the leaflet and understood the implications of being a donor.

## Semen donation

Although the number of samples a donor will give must be his decision, we do tell our donors that all being well, we would like somewhere in the region of 50 samples. All samples must be produced on the licensed premises of the bank. Donors ask at the laboratory for the correct sample jar which is then marked with his initials or code number. He then goes to one of the rooms provided to produce his sample. It is necessary for adequate toilet facilities to be provided as personal hygiene is very important. This fact must be stressed during the counselling session. Our donors are not allowed to supply more than two samples in any one week, and should the quality of their donation be below the required standard, the interval of production is increased. A small sum of money is paid on receipt of the sample to cover expenses. Some centres will pay half at the time of production and the rest when the donor returns later for the repeat screening tests. Although we do not allow more than two samples in any one week, we do not state a number that must be produced each week. Should it be convenient for a donor to supply one sample a week or even only one a month, that is acceptable. No donor should be pressured into producing samples at more frequent intervals than is comfortable.

## Filing and coding

There are many methods of filing and coding donor records, and each establishment will adopt a method suited to their equipment and facilities; however the less complicated a system is, the less is the risk of confusion and mistakes. The method that we have used for the past 20 years has, so far, not let us down. After acceptance into the programme each donor is given a code number which is derived by using the prefix A, B, O or AB according to their blood group, followed by the numerical order in which they applied to become semen donors. Therefore the first Group A donor would be A1 followed by his rhesus status, i.e. A1POS. Should the second donor to apply have the blood group A and is rhesus negative, his code becomes A2NEG.

## Cryoprotectant

Glycerol, which is a permeating cryoprotectant, is the most popular component of cryoprotectant mixtures for semen freezing. Although egg yolk is not a cryoprotectant it appears to help stabilise the sperm membrane thereby maintaining its fluidity. Citrate and glycine are used as pH buffers for the mixture. There are now many commercial preparations suitable for semen freezing but

Table 12.2. *Constituents of GEYC medium*

| Component | Quantity |
| --- | --- |
| 3% Tri-sodium citrate | 39 ml |
| 5.5% Glucose solution | 26 ml |
| Glycerol | 15 ml |
| Egg yolk (filtered through gauze) | 20 ml |
| Glycine | 1.5 g |
| Erythromycin | 0.1 g |
| Total volume | 100 ml |

*Notes:*
GEYC: glycerol/egg yolk/citrate

we still prefer to prepare our cryoprotectant solution on site and we use a glycerol/egg yolk/citrate medium (Table 12.2) first described by Matheson *et al.* (1969). This is simple to make and is very economical. All solutions are made with tissue culture grade sterile water. Tri-sodium citrate, glucose solution, glycerol and egg yolk are mixed together before adding glycine and erythromycin and mixing again. The solution is then incubated at 56 °C for 30 minutes and cooled to room temperature. The pH is adjusted to within the range of 7.2–7.4 using a weak solution of sodium bicarbonate. This makes 100 ml of cryoprotectant solution which is best stored in 20 ml aliquots away from light in the refrigerator. Any sample that will be stored for more than 1 week should be put in the freezer compartment.

### Addition of cryoprotectant to semen

The semen sample is allowed to stand on the bench for about 30 minutes after production for complete liquefaction to take place. A routine analysis is carried out to confirm adequacy of the semen parameters. The volume of the semen sample is accurately measured as an equal volume of cryoprotectant solution will be added to it. The cryoprotectant is added drop-wise to the semen sample while gently swirling around the sample to ensure proper mixing. The mixture is allowed to stand for 15 minutes at room temperature before using negative pressure to fill appropriate straws and seal with polyvinyl alcohol (PVA) powder.

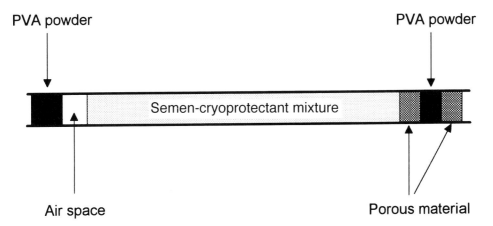

Figure 12.1. Straw filled with semen-cryoprotectant mixture.

### Packaging

The semen-cryoprotectant mixture is placed in small (0.25 ml) plastic straws and PVA powder is used as a seal. The straws come in assorted colours as does the PVA powder. This means that the straws and seal can be used in identifying different donors. At present we use 11 different colours of straws and eight different PVA powder colours. This gives 88 colour combinations to use in filing and coding donor samples. A straw will already contain a porous plug at one end and the centre of this plug will have a small amount of PVA powder in situ (Figure 12.1). A plastic is formed as soon as moisture comes in contact with the PVA powder thereby creating a watertight seal. After being filled with the semen-cryoprotectant mixture the open end of the straw is sealed with the coloured PVA powder. The straw is then ready for the freezing process. We do not encourage the use of glass ampoules for cryopreservation as they tend to explode during thawing and may constitute a source of danger to staff and contaminate other patients' samples. Plastic cryovials may not allow efficient cooling of the whole sample although the use of vials with conical base and vanes may improve the heat transfer (Mortimer 1994). Furthermore, the volume of fluid in the vial should not exceed 1 ml. A major advantage of using straws is that a large number of them can be stored in one dewer and this is an important consideration in units that handle a large number of samples such as ours.

### Freezing method

Many banks would have developed their own or adapted methods of freezing that suit their own establishment and equipment. We advocate the use of

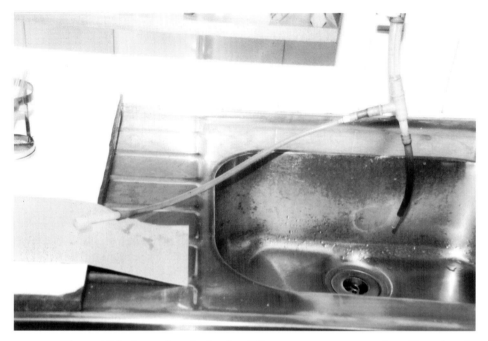

Figure 12.2. A suction device for filling many straws at a time. Running the water tap will create negative pressure in the system which draws the semen-cryoprotectant mixture into the straws that are attached to the suction head.

simple, reliable methods that provide consistently good results. This is associated with less likelihood of machinery breakdown or failure. We use a static vapour phase cooling method and suspend the straws in liquid nitrogen vapour for 15–30 minutes. This will give the required temperature fall of approximately 7 °C per minute, to −70 °C. The straws are then plunged into liquid nitrogen and stored at that temperature (−196 °C) until the time they are required. While stored in this way minimal deterioration occurs, and frozen sperms are still viable for at least 10 years, and longer. Key steps in the freezing procedure and subsequent storage are shown in Figures 12.2–12.7.

### Storage of frozen semen

Once a donor has been accepted in a programme, an efficient and reliable storage and filing system must be used. No donor semen is frozen and stored until the initial screening results are received. If these tests are negative, the donor produces samples which are frozen and stored in liquid nitrogen dewers reserved for quarantined donors. If the second screen, which is carried out 7 months later, is negative, these samples can then be put into use. Relevant

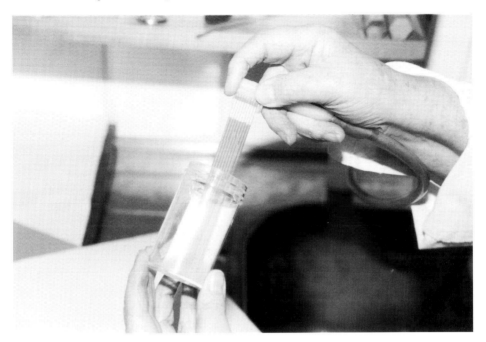

Figure 12.3. Several straws being filled at a time with the semen-cryoprotectant mixture.

details of these quarantined samples can be displayed at a prominent part of the laboratory to make it easier for staff to monitor the progress from quarantine to use (Figure 12.8). It is also important that infection screening is carried out regularly. If positive tests result at any time all samples from that donor should be discarded and no further freezing should take place. If all tests are negative and continue to be so the frozen samples may be used until ten pregnancies have been achieved (in the UK). It is also advisable whenever possible to keep some frozen samples in storage after the ten allowed births for use by couples wishing for siblings from the same donor. Again filing and storage must be such that samples from donors who have reached the permitted quota of pregnancies must not be in a tank where it could inadvertently be used for other than to conceive a sibling.

Each time a new batch of semen is frozen, a post-thaw analysis of sperm survival is carried out the following day on a sample from one of the frozen straws. The post-thaw recovery must be of sufficient numbers to be viable for use in artificial insemination; each 0.25 ml straw must contain at least three million live spermatozoa showing good motility and progressive movement. If the post-thaw recovery is less than required all the straws from that batch of semen are discarded. Frozen samples from each donor are kept in small goblets

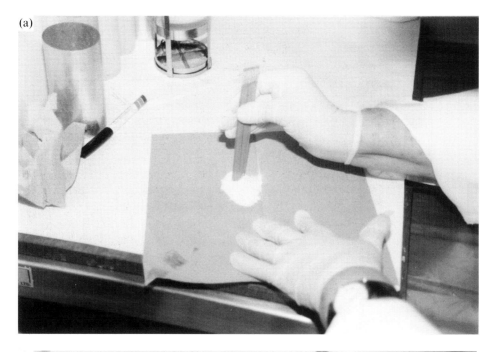

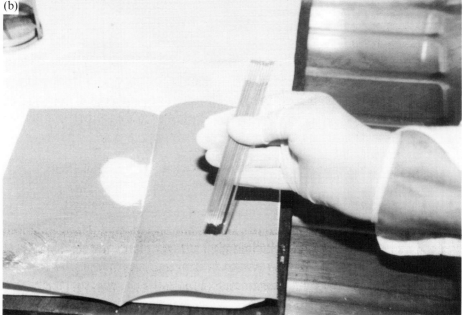

Figure 12.4. Fluid is displaced from the lower ends of the straws with a comb-like device followed by tamping in polyvinyl alcohol powder which solidifies on contact with moisture, thereby sealing that end of the straws.

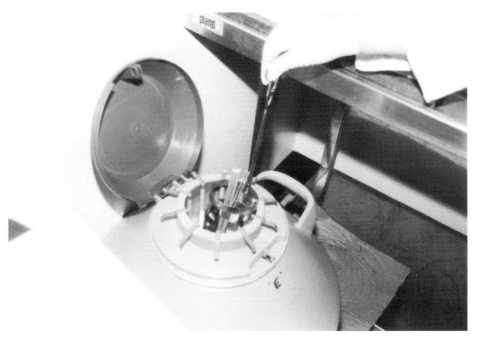

Figure 12.5. Filled straws are loaded in a metal basket and suspended in liquid nitrogen vapour.

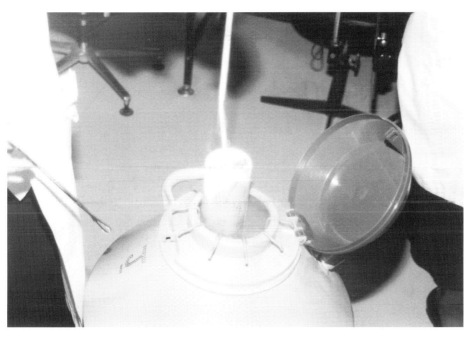

Figure 12.6. The frozen samples are transferred into goblets which are placed in the metal cannister for storage in liquid nitrogen containing dewers.

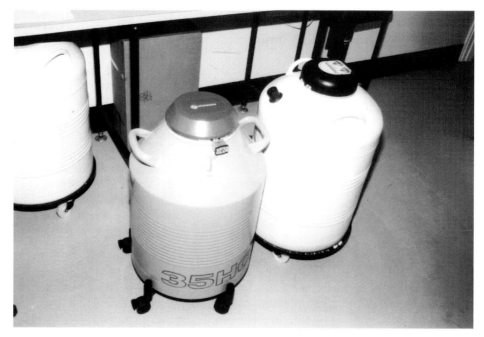

Figure 12.7. Each dewer in the unit must be identified with a unique mark, name or combination of alphabets and numbers.

labelled with the donor code number, the colour of the straws and seal together with the month and year it was frozen and stored. This enables accurate movement and subsequent checks of each donor's straws as and when the initial quarantine period is over. It is advisable not to store more than 500 straws from any one donor. This is because the allowed ten pregnancies could be reached before many straws have been released into circulation leading to loss of the substantial capital outlay. A bank could find itself in a position where it has numerous surplus straws that have to be discarded.

### Matching donor-recipient characteristics

It is extremely important to record non-identifying donor characteristics which will be used in assisting selection of donor semen for patients. Information commonly supplied include the donor's ethnic origin, blood group, hair and eye colour, complexion, height, build, profession, interests and hobbies. Similar information from the recipient and her husband will enable as close a match as possible to be made. It should be stated clearly whether the blood groups should be matched or not. Particular note has to be taken in Rhesus negative women as a Rhesus positive foetus will increase the chances of her

# Donor sperm banking

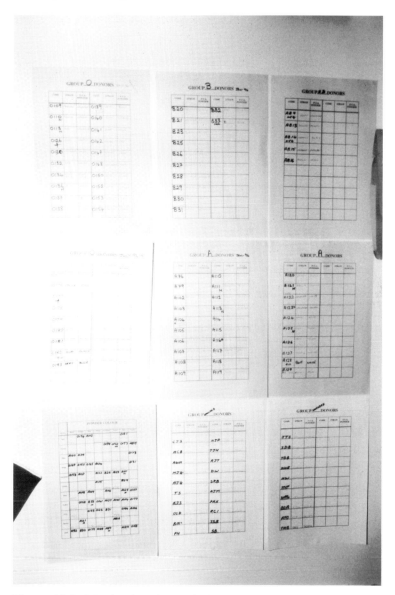

Figure 12.8. Monitoring the period of quarrantine of stored semen can be made easier by display of relevant details at a prominent place in the laboratory.

becoming sensitised against the Rhesus positive blood cells unless proper prophylactic measures are taken.

### Insemination

For direct artificial insemination it would be advisable to use at least two straws, and for washed and concentrated samples for intrauterine insemination, four straws would be more realistic. About three million motile spermatozoa per straw is the very least one would expect from a frozen semen sample. A more common recovery is however ten million motile spermatozoa. Artificial insemination should always be timed by efficient and accurate ovulation screening techniques. If ovulation is found to be erratic, irregular or even non-existent, then appropriate hormonal or ovulation induction treatment is usually prescribed.

### Conclusion

A donor sperm bank is an asset to any fertility treatment centre. Unless the centre carries out more than 150 donor inseminations a year, it is probably more cost-effective to procure donor semen from other banks than setting up a new one. Frozen semen is easily transferred over long distances with dry-shippers (Figure 12.9). Donor semen is likely to be required for a long time to come. Some uncommon indications such as insemination of single women or lesbians may become more common place in future as societal norms undergo modification. The highest standards should be maintained in these banks so as to protect all parties affected by the activities taking place there. This includes observance of health and safety measures (Figure 12.10). There should be more research aimed at finding out better freezing techniques which will be associated with improved cryosurvival of sperm and increased pregnancy rates.

### References

Barratt C. L. R., Matson P. L. & Holt W. (1993) British Andrology Society guidelines for the screening of semen donors for donor insemination. *Human Reproduction* **8**, 1521–1523.

Matheson G.W., Carlborg L. & Gemzell C. (1969) Frozen human semen for artificial insemination. *American Journal of Obstetrics and Gynecology* **104**, 495–501.

Mortimer D. (1994) Semen cryopreservation. In: *Practical Laboratory Andrology*. Oxford Universtiy Press, New York. pp. 301–323.

World Health Organization (1992) *WHO laboratory manual for the examination of human semen and sperm-cervical mucus interaction,* third edition. Cambridge University Press, Cambridge.

## Donor sperm banking

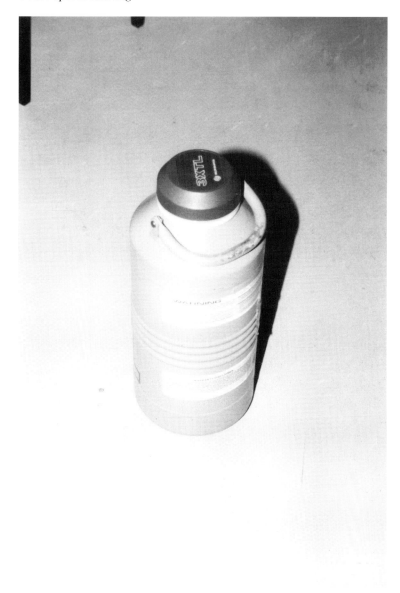

Figure 12.9. A dry-shipper such as the one shown here makes it possible for assisted conception units to be supplied with frozen semen by banks that are far away from the units.

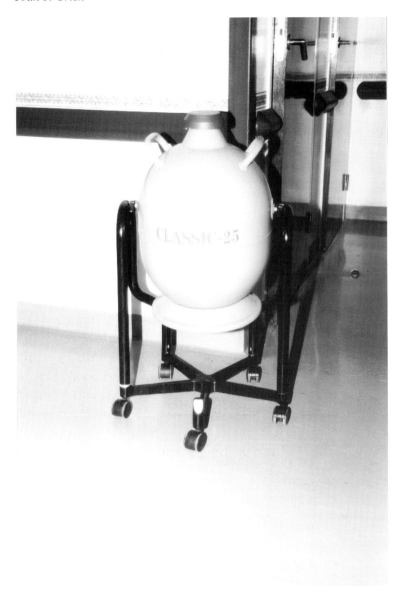

Figure 12.10. The chances of staff sustaining back injury causing accidental spillage of liquid nitrogen can be minimised by having a specially mounted dewer which can be used for moving liquid nitrogen from one part of the unit to the other.

# 13

# Complications of superovulation and intrauterine insemination

GODWIN I. MENIRU

### Introduction

Intrauterine insemination (IUI) is one of the least invasive of all assisted conception treatments. Consequently, complications are uncommon but this fact actually makes it imperative for the practitioner to become familiar with details of the few problems. This will ensure that the low incidence profile is maintained as well as aiding the early recognition of their occurrence and provide effective treatment. Complications may arise as a result of the insemination procedure itself or be related to other interventions during the treatment of these women, such as superovulation. Side-effects of the orally administered medications, clomiphene citrate, cyclofenil and tamoxifen, are shown in Table 13.1. The rest of this chapter will be dedicated to discussions on other problems that can be encountered during fertility treatment with IUI.

### Ovarian hyperstimulation syndrome

Ovarian hyperstimulation syndrome (OHSS) is usually found in females who have had induction of ovulation or superovulation. It consists of ovarian enlargement and pathologies arising from an acute fluid shift out of the intravascular compartment and into the potential spaces (Table 13.2). Its incidence and severity vary depending on the presence of risk factors (Table 13.3). The incidence is much lower when clomiphene citrate is used in comparison to administration of gonadotrophins, and the advent of gonadotrophin releasing hormone agonists (GnRHa) has not led to a fall in the incidence. In fact the incidence of OHSS is highest in cycles employing GnRHa (Tan 1994). This may be because the premature luteinising hormone surge, which is probably one of the body's protective mechanisms against excessive ovarian activity, is

Table 13.1. *Side-effects of orally administered ovulation induction agents*

|  | Clomiphene | Cyclofenil | Tamoxifen |
|---|---|---|---|
| Hot flushes | ✓ | ✓ | ✓ |
| Nausea | ✓ | ✓ | ✓ |
| Abdominal discomfort | ✓ | ✓ |  |
| Weight gain | ✓ |  | ✓ |
| Vomiting | ✓ |  | ✓ |
| Dizziness | ✓ |  | ✓ |
| Depression | ✓ |  |  |
| Visual disturbances | ✓ |  |  |
| Ovarian hyperstimulation | ✓ |  |  |
| Insomnia | ✓ |  |  |
| Breast tenderness | ✓ |  |  |
| Rashes | ✓ |  |  |
| Hair loss | ✓ |  |  |
| Cholestatic jaundice |  | ✓ |  |
| Menstrual disturbances |  |  | ✓ |
| Acne |  |  | ✓ |
| Headaches |  |  | ✓ |

*Source:* British National Formulary (1994); Taubert and Kuhl (1993)

abolished by these analogues. Previously, detection of this premature hormone surge could have meant cancellation of the treatment cycle.

Earlier systems of classification of OHSS were based on clinical and laboratory criteria (Rabau *et al.* 1967; Schenker & Weinstein 1978) but Golan *et al.* (1989) proposed a system that is based mainly on clinical and ultrasound features (Table 13.4). This is especially relevant to the current practice in many centres of not using hormone assays to monitor stimulation cycles. Some degree of OHSS is found in 25% or more of patients having superovulation for in vitro fertilisation (IVF) but this is mainly of the mild variety. Severe OHSS occurs usually in less than 2% of patients although it may reach 10% at times (references in Rizk 1992). The incidence is lower in IUI cycles due to the relatively smaller doses of administered gonadotrophins. OHSS has been estimated to occur in 1% of IUI cycles although the incidence increases in conceptual cycles (Dodson & Haney 1991; Ombelet *et al.* 1995a). The reported incidence of OHSS varies because many centres differ in their approach to superovulation, classification of OHSS and intensity of patient follow up. It is likely that many cases of mild and some of moderate OHSS are missed as contact with the patient is less in the luteal phase than during the period of fol-

Table 13.2. *Spectrum of disorders in ovarian hyperstimulation syndrome*

Ovarian enlargement
Ascites
Pleural effusion
Hydrothorax
Haemoconcentration
Electrolyte disturbances
Coagulation defects and thromboembolism
Liver dysfunction
Renal disorders (decreased renal perfusion and oliguria)
Torsion of the ovary
Cerebrovascular accident
Adult respiratory distress syndrome

Table 13.3. *Risk factors for the development of ovarian hyperstimulation syndrome*

Age less than 35 years
Polycystic ovaries
Type of superovulation agents used and their dose
Conception in the index treatment cycle
Previous history of OHSS
Serum oestradiol concentration exceeding 10000 pmol/l before hCG injection
Rapid increase in oestradiol concentration during follicular stimulation
Large number (>15–20) of small and medium sized follicles (12–14 mm)

*Notes:*
hCG: human chorionic gonadotrophin; OHSS: ovarian hyperstimulation syndrome.

licular stimulation. Much of the following information on OHSS has been gathered from IVF rather than IUI cycles. It is however necessary to include it here so as to provide a comprehensive account that will be very useful to the reader who is not a subspecialist in reproductive medicine.

No one knows exactly how OHSS arises but the acute fluid shift out of the intravascular compartment is due to increased capillary permeability. Hormones and other compounds that have been investigated include oestrogen, progesterone, testosterone, prostaglandins, histamine, prolactin, inhibin, serotonin, aldosterone, products of the ovarian renin–angiotensin system, CA-125, cytokines and platelet-derived growth factor. None of these has been

Table 13.4. *Classification of ovarian hyperstimulation syndrome*

| Grade | Clinical features and findings |
|---|---|
| *Mild* | |
| 1 | Abdominal distension and discomfort |
| 2 | (1) + nausea, vomiting and/or diarrhoea; enlarged ovaries (5–12 cm) |
| *Moderate* | |
| 3 | Features of mild OHSS + ascites seen on ultrasound scan |
| *Severe* | |
| 4 | Features of moderate OHSS + ascites diagnosed clinically and/or hydrothorax and breathing difficulties |
| 5 | (1) to (4) + haemoconcentration, coagulopathy and diminished renal perfusion and function |

*Notes:*
OHSS: ovarian hyperstimulation syndrome

clearly shown to have a categorical role in the pathogenesis of OHSS. Although other agents may be involved, human chorionic gonadotrophin (hCG) appears to play a pivotal role in the pathogenesis of this complication since OHSS occurs almost exclusively in cycles in which hCG has been administered or is being produced endogenously by the early conceptus. OHSS seems to have two varieties that differ mainly in their temporal relationship to administration of the ovulatory dose of hCG (Amso 1995). The 'early presentation' type manifests within 7 days of the hCG injection while the 'late presentation' type presents between 12 and 17 days following the injection and is caused by endogenous hCG production by the conceptus. It is also possible for early manifestations of OHSS to persist or even worsen if conception takes place in that cycle. Clinical features of OHSS include evidence of decreased intravascular volume such as hypotension, low central venous pressure and tachycardia (Tsirigotis & Craft 1994). Varying degrees of abdominal distension with discomfort may be present depending on the extent of ovarian enlargement and ascites (Table 13.4). Some patients may manifest with respiratory embarrassment, coagulation defects, hepatic disorders and renal failure. Death is a real possibility in very severe cases if not managed appropriately.

Prevention begins with identification of groups of patients at risk of having OHSS (Table 13.3) and modifying the superovulation regimen so as to achieve the right balance between optimal response and excessive follicular development. The syndrome can however develop unexpectedly at times. Development of an excessive number (> 15) of small to medium sized (12–14 mm) follicles during stimulation, with enlarged ovaries of more than 5 cm in diameter, are warning signs. Symptoms of nausea, lower abdominal pain and distension before hCG administration are evidence of the development of the severe form of OHSS. If serum oestradiol assay is available, concentrations of over 10 000 pmol/L and rising are strong warning signs too.

The dosage of gonadotrophins administered early in the cycle should be reduced once monitoring indicates a risk. Changing the ovulation triggering hormone from hCG to GnRHa has been suggested as another way to reduce the risk and severity when a GnRHa is not included in the superovulation regimen (Gonen *et al.* 1990). An example is buserelin (Suprefact; Hoechst UK Ltd, Hounslow, UK) which can be administered subcutaneously as a single dose of 1 mg. Intravenous infusion of hyperoncotic human albumin solution (Human Albumin Solution 20% BP Immuno; Immuno AG, Vienna, Austria) at the time of oocyte aspiration in IVF treatment cycles can also reduce the risk and severity (Asch *et al.* 1993; Shahata *et al.* 1994; Shoham *et al.* 1994). Similar principles may apply to IUI cycles in which case, the infusion is administered at the time of insemination; however it may be more appropriate to consider alternative treatment strategies, such as the following, if the risk of OHSS seems real enough to justify this infusion, when a patient is assessed in the late follicular phase of an IUI treatment cycle.

The treatment modality may be changed from IUI to IVF or gamete intrafallopian transfer (GIFT) as this affords the opportunity to empty all developing follicles. Repeated aspiration and flushing of follicles decreases the granulosa cell content of these follicles and this may reduce the incidence and severity of OHSS (Waterstone *et al.* 1991) although this assertion has been challenged by Wada *et al.* (1993a). The real benefit of the change from IUI to IVF is that all resulting embryos can be cryopreserved and transferred in a subsequent frozen embryo replacement cycle. Even though this may not completely prevent OHSS, the severity and period of debility is decreased when there is no endogenous production of hCG by an early conceptus (Wada *et al.* 1993b). The absence of pregnancy will also allow more leeway for the use of pharmacological agents such as angiotensin converting enzyme inhibitor without fear of teratogenicity (Brinsden *et al.* 1995). Elective embryo cryopreservation is an appropriate measure as evidenced by an embryo survival rate of 72% on thawing and a clinical pregnancy rate of 26% per embryo transfer cycle (Wada *et al.* 1992).

Another preventive measure is that of withholding the ovulatory hCG injection and abandoning the treatment cycle (Forman *et al.* 1990). The dose of superovulation agents is decreased in subsequent cycles in a bid to avoid repetition of the same problem of impending OHSS. Some workers have found that this approach is associated with poor ovarian responses in these repeat cycles as the understandably cautious clinician often administers insufficient doses of gonadotrophins and many unsatisfactory treatment cycles may be conducted in this manner (Amso *et al.* 1991; Wada *et al.* 1993a). Following cancellation of a treatment cycle because of the fear of provoking OHSS, the couple should be advised to abstain from sexual intercourse for 2 or more weeks. This is because spontaneous ovulation can occur during that period if GnRHa is discontinued. Conception with a resulting severe OHSS has been reported in such circumstances (Lipitz *et al.* 1991). It may be more prudent to continue GnRHa administration until complete follicular regression occurs. The patient may in fact go on to a fresh treatment cycle without stopping GnRHa administration that was commenced in the preceding cancelled cycle. If a decision is made to continue with a superovulation cycle in which there is a risk of OHSS the normal ovulatory dose of hCG (10000 IU) may be halved and luteal phase support provided with progesterone instead of hCG (Tsirigotis & Craft 1994). The use of steroids or antihistamines has not been shown to be of proven benefit in preventing the occurrence of OHSS.

Treatment of OHSS depends on its severity, amongst other considerations. If it is mild or moderate and the haematocrit is equal to or less than 44% (Amso 1995), treatment is carried out on an outpatient basis unless the condition of the patient worsens. The patient should be treated with bedrest and increased fluid, and have regular haematological and biochemical screening tests (Amso 1995). Analgesics and anti-emetics may be required in some cases but worsening of the patient's symptoms suggests the need for careful re-evaluation and possibly hospital admission. Regular ultrasound scans are also necessary to confirm steady improvement of the condition.

If severe OHSS develops, it is important that it is recognised early; hence patients at risk need to be monitored 3–4 days after the insemination and regularly afterwards, if required. Development of nausea, vomiting, abdominal pain, dyspnea and marked distension indicates OHSS of moderate severity that needs treatment. Ultrasound may show enlarged ovaries of > 7 cm each and the presence of ascites (Figure 13.1). In-patient treatment is required for those with severe OHSS or where there is worsening of the moderate type. It is advisable for the patient's treatment to be carried out by a specialist who has experience in treating OHSS, with backup cover being provided by intensive (critical) care specialists. A number of investigations should be performed on admission (Table 13.5) and repeated at appropriate intervals as dictated by the patient's condition. Treatment is aimed at restoration of the normal plasma volume and maintenance of renal perfusion while waiting for spontaneous resolution of the condition. Intravenous infusion of crystalloids and colloids is performed to correct the electrolyte imbalance and re-expand the plasma volume. The use of hyperoncotic human albumin infusion will help draw fluid back into the circulation from the extravascular compartment as well as correct the existing hypoalbuminaemia. There is need for insertion of a central venous pressure line in patients with severe OHSS (Brinsden *et al.* 1995). Administration of antiplatelet drugs such as aspirin or dipyridamole, or anticoagulants (heparin) is commenced if there is evidence of coagulopathy or thromboembolism but this decision should be made in consultation with a haematologist. There is as yet no unanimity on the efficacy of various other drugs that have been proposed for use in cases of severe OHSS (Table 13.6).

It is not likely that paracentesis will be required in a case of OHSS following superovulation for IUI because of the expected low severity of the problem. Marked distension of the abdomen by ascitic fluid to the extent that it causes respiratory embarrassment or is associated with failing renal function justifies this procedure which should be carried out transabdominally or transvaginally under ultrasound guidance. Dramatic improvement in the patient's condition and urine output tends to follow this procedure (Tsirigotis & Craft 1994; Amso 1995) and paracentesis thoracis is usually not required after this. Surgery is seldom required and should only be embarked upon for clearly recognised indications such as haemorrhage, torsion of the ovary and ruptured ovarian cysts (Amso 1995). A conservative approach should be adopted; haemostasis is secured in cases of haemorrhage from the ovary and the abdomen closed. Untwisting of the torsion should be tried first and this may be the only required surgical manoeuvre in many patients with this problem (Mashiach *et al.* 1990). A rare indication for surgery in women with severe OHSS is a coexisting ectopic pregnancy. Similarly, termination of the pregnancy is rarely required except in the case of a patient with very severe OHSS that is unresponsive to other treatment.

## Multiple pregnancy

Superovulation and IUI aim at increasing gamete density at the natural site of fertilisation in the fallopian tubes to overcome fertility dysfunction in couples. Usually, production of three and not more than four fertilisable oocytes is the goal but there is no way of confirming that this number is not exceeded in some cases. This is because smaller sized follicles, which are not taken into account at the time of administering the ovulatory dose of hCG, may still yield viable oocytes. These will swell the pool of fertilisable oocytes picked up by the tubes following ovulation. There may be improper monitoring of superovulation or none at all. It is also not possible to predict the fertilisation rate of ovulated

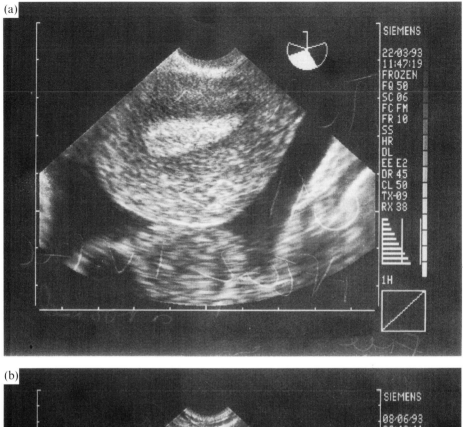

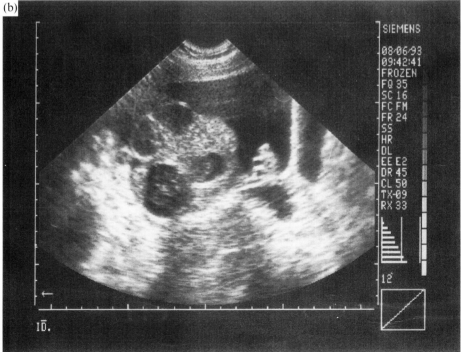

Figure 13.1. Ultrasound features of severe ovarian hyperstimulation syndrome. There is marked ascites, with fluid surrounding various organs in the

(c)

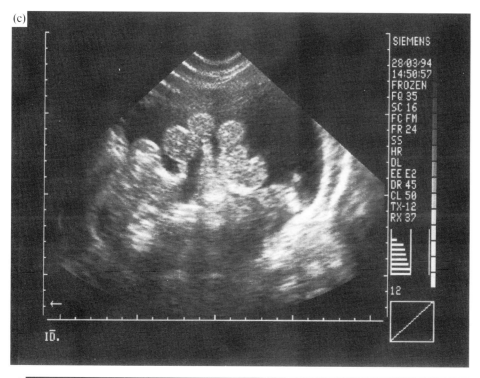

(d)

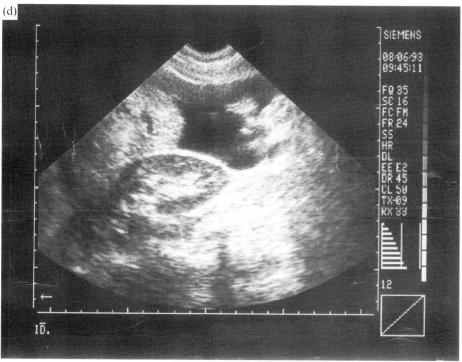

abdomen and pelvis: (a) uterus, (b) ovary, (c) bowel loops, and (d) liver and kidney.

Table 13.5. *Assessment of patients with severe ovarian hyperstimulation syndrome*

---

Fluid balance chart
Daily measurement of abdominal girth and body weight
Full blood count, especially haematocrit
Serum electrolytes, urea and creatinine
Serum albumin and total protein
Liver function tests
Abdominal and pelvic ultrasound scans
Clotting studies
Serum and urine osmolarity
Chest X-ray
Central venous pressure
Pregnancy test (2 weeks after embryo transfer)

---

Table 13.6. *Treatment of severe ovarian hyperstimulation syndrome*

---

*Established treatment modality*
Correction of electrolyte imbalance with crystalloids
Plasma expansion with colloid solutions such as albumin
Paracentesis
Other supportive therapy
Anticoagulants if indicated

*Treatment of unproven benefit*
Antihistamines
Prostaglandin synthetase inhibitors (e.g. indomethacin)
Danazol
Gonadotrophin releasing hormone agonist

---

oocytes and the subsequent implantation rate in each cycle of treatment. Multiple pregnancy is a common problem after IUI just as in most other assisted conception treatment techniques but its incidence varies widely. The multiple pregnancy rate in a retrospective review of 1100 IUI cycles was found to be 11.4% (17 out of 149 pregnancies) by Ombelet et al. (1995b). Out of the 17 multiple pregnancies, 15 were twin while the other two were triplet pregnancies. Higher multiple pregnancy rates of up to 30% have been found in other studies.

Multiple pregnancy is associated with a significantly higher incidence of

Table 13.7. *The problems of multiple pregnancy*

Hyperemesis gravidarum
Anaemia
Pre-eclampsia
Varicose veins
Pedal oedema
Dyspepsia
Miscarriage
Polyhydramnios
Antepartum haemorrhage
Pre-term labour and delivery
Premature rupture of membranes
Cord accidents
Intrauterine growth retardation
Malpresentation and abnormal lie
Post-partum haemorrhage
Caesarean delivery
Foetal abnormality
Stillbirth

complications (Table 13.7) leading to increase in foetal loss, maternal morbidity, perinatal morbidity and mortality, when compared to singleton pregnancies. Preterm delivery is particularly common especially in higher order multiple pregnancies (triplets and above). Management of the preterm infant often involves prolonged care in neonatal intensive care units and is very expensive to the state which usually bears the cost of such services. Survivors may have residual deficits which require further care and rehabilitation in the community. Some disabilities may even render them totally dependent on others for sustenance for the rest of their lives. Many families thus may find it difficult coping with the emotional, social, economic and physical stress which this situation imposes on them.

The multiple pregnancy rate is significantly higher in IUI cycles in which gonadotrophins are administered when compared to those using clomiphene citrate alone for superovulation (Ombelet *et al.* 1995a). As expected the pregnancy rate is also higher in the former cycles. This underscores the predicament that often faces the practitioner regarding the agent and dose to be used, hence the number of preovulatory follicles to recruit and nurture till ovulation. On one hand, the clinician, and patient too, would like to maximise the chances of conception by inducing multiple follicular development while on the other hand, all parties do wish and aim for the lowest possible multiple pregnancy rate. Part of the solution lies in the formulation of a prognostic index that will include such parameters as the patient's age, build, cause and duration of infertility, number of previous IUI cycles, previous response to superovulation, and so on. This will assist the clinician to decide on the optimal strategy for ovarian stimulation. At present even the most careful approach to superovulation and cycle monitoring with ultrasonography and hormone assays cannot guarantee avoidance of multiple pregnancy especially when gonadotrophins are used (Ombelet et al. 1995b). Surprisingly, some workers have reported that the risk of multiple pregnancy may not depend, as previously thought, on the number of mature follicles (> 16 mm) developing or the quality of sperm, but can be quite unpredictable (Friedman et al. 1992).

A number of management options can be considered if ovarian response to superovulation for IUI is in excess of expectation. Aspiration of supernumerary follicles may be carried out prior to IUI but a change of treatment to IVF or GIFT at this time is a better option and needs to be discussed carefully with the couple. This is because it will allow more precise control over the number of embryos or eggs transferred. Abandoning the treatment and withholding the ovulatory injection of hCG should also be discussed. If higher order multiple pregnancy occurs selective foetocide (foetal reduction) under ultrasound control may be the only realistic means of managing this problem but the emotional and/or moral dilemma this presents to many couples has to be appreciated. Counselling and proper support should be provided to these couples but perhaps the best approach should be to avoid placing these vulnerable individuals in such a predicament by adopting a more careful approach to superovulation for IUI.

### Ovarian cancer?

The possibility of an association between ovarian stimulation and ovarian cancer was raised by Fishel and Jackson in 1989. They discussed three hypotheses regarding the aetiology of ovarian cancers in such circumstances: (1) the effect of multiple ovulations in disrupting the ovarian epithelium which ultimately leads to malignant transformation, (2) persistent ovarian stimulation by gonadotrophins which may act alone or in concert with oestrogens, and (3) gonadotrophin/steroid-induced metabolism of chemical carcinogens (also called xenobiotics) such as 7, 12-dimethylbenz (a) anthracene in the ovary. Reactive intermediates of these compounds may cause destruction of follicular cells or induce their malignant transformation. These pioneer workers then went on to review three published case reports of ovarian cancer in three women aged 25, 26 and 32 years, respectively. It is worthy of note that presentation of these tumours was acute, following superovulation with large doses of clomiphene citrate or gonadotrophins.

There have been more case reports since that paper including that of Willemsen *et al.* (1993) who presented 12 cases in support of a possible link between ovarian stimulation and granulosa cell tumour. These authors discussed three possibilities; (1) the granulosa cell tumour is present in the ovary and the hormonal stimulus accelerates its clinical manifestation, (2) increased follicle stimulating hormone concentration is oncogenic to granulosa cells, and (3) the appearance of a granulosa cell tumour during ovarian stimulation is coincidental. This writer is aware of another patient with granulosa cell tumour who was managed by a senior colleague. She was a 35 year old woman with primary infertility and oligomenorrhoea and presented with a left sided pelvic mass, confirmed by ultrasound scanning, after three cycles of ovulation induction with 100 mg of clomiphene citrate. This mass measured 13 cm by 11 cm and contained multiple solid and cystic areas. Her serum oestradiol concentration was 5734 pmol/L. Left salpingo-oophorectomy was performed and a histological diagnosis of granulosa cell tumour made. Her serum oestradiol concentration 6 weeks after surgery was 363 pmol/L and regular menstrual periods resumed shortly afterwards. Findings in this case lend support to the hypothesis that the tumour predates ovarian stimulation, its rapid growth and clinical presentation being triggered off by an increased level of gonadotrophins. This patient was noted to have had unilateral ovarian enlargement before the first cycle of ovarian stimulation. An irregularly shaped follicle in the left ovary might have been the early tumour. There was subsequently marked and rapid enlargement of that ovary after treatment with clomiphene citrate. Spontaneous return of regular menstrual periods after the operation provides further circumstantial evidence to support this line of thought and has been noted by others (Lappohn *et al.* 1989; Willemsen *et al.* 1993)

A number of studies have now been carried out which while not establishing a causal relationship have not dispelled the fear that there might be some sort of association between some cases of ovarian cancer and prior ovulation induction or superovulation (Harris *et al.* 1992; Horn-Ross *et al.* 1992; Whittemore *et al.* 1992). These reports were based on the results of a combined analysis of data from previous case control studies. The reliability of these studies has been challenged on a number of points that revolve around the design and completeness of the data (Balasch & Barri 1993; Cohen *et al.* 1993). As Whittemore (1993) pointed out in a rejoinder, the correct attitude of the medical and scientific community at this moment should be that of continuing endeavours to find out more about this (nebulous) association and not that of discrediting present evidence on the grounds of faulty research methodology. The idea that ovarian stimulation may cause ovarian cancer is not far fetched and should not be treated as such.

Subsequent reports (Rossing *et al.* 1994; Venn *et al.* 1995; Shushan *et al.* 1996) have not removed this uncertainty. Rather they provide evidence that indicates a greater chance of ovarian and possibly other female tumours arising in infertile women who have had assisted conception treatment involving superovulation. Shushan *et al.* (1996) accessed the Israel Cancer Registry to obtain the names of patients who were reported to have had ovarian cancer. Those who were still alive were later interviewed to ascertain their obstetric and gynaecological history with special emphasis on infertility and fertility treatment. This group was then compared to a group of randomly selected women and the results showed that epithelial ovarian cancers were three times more likely to develop in patients who had had previous treatment with gonadotrophins. There was also a strong association between gonadotrophin administration and borderline ovarian tumours (OR 9.38, 95% CI 1.66 to 52.08) (Shushan *et al.* 1996). Venn and colleagues (1995) compared infertile women who had had superovulation and IVF, with those who were referred for IVF but ended up not having any treatment at all or had treatment that did not involve ovarian stimulation. These groups were also compared with the general female population. They found that the incidence of breast cancer was not higher in women who had had ovarian stimulation but that of ovarian cancer was higher when all women who had been referred for IVF treatment were compared to the general population. The increase in incidence of ovarian cancer was however not statistically significant. A significant increase in the incidence of uterine cancer was found when these infertile women were compared to the general population. Interestingly, ovarian and uterine cancers were more closely associated with unexplained infertility than any other aetiology of infertility.

Cancer is a multifactorial disease and it would be naive to believe or seek a simple relationship between infertility and its treatment on the one hand and the genesis of malignancy on the other hand. If ovarian stimulants are later proven to have a role in the development of malignancy in women it is likely to be complex, involving several intermediary pathways and modulators including genetic and environmental factors (Figure 13.2). The fact that the large majority of females who undergo ovulation induction or superovulation do not develop malignancy gives credence to this speculation. Review of published reports show that there may be two classes of effects of ovarian stimulation. An early effect takes the form of unmasking an existing tumour by

Complications

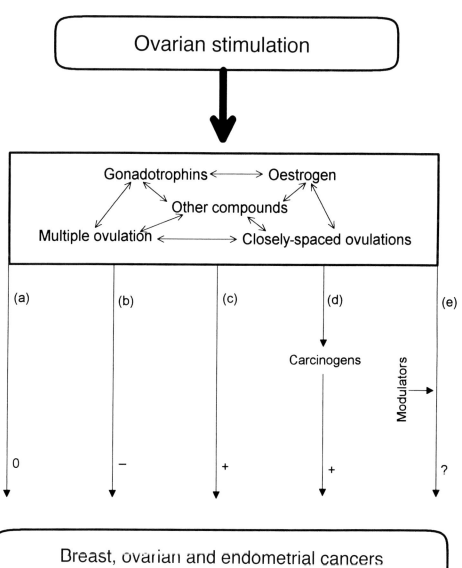

Figure 13.2. Possible relationships of ovarian stimulation to the pathogenesis of some cancers in females. (a) No effect at all; (b) negative (protective) effect; (c) direct positive (enhancing) effect; (d) indirect positive effect mediated through elaboration of carcinogens; (e) uncertain effect; depends on interaction with modulators such as type and duration of infertility, genetic influences, environmental and lifestyle factors, oral contraceptive usage, pregnancies, breast feeding, ovulatory age and so on.

accelerating its clinical manifestation through a hormonally driven increase in vascular supply to the affected organ or a direct effect on cell growth. This may explain the appearance of some cancers during ovarian stimulation or soon afterwards. The late effect takes many years to manifest and will constitute what actually is the real oncogenic action of ovarian stimulants. Epidemiological data and prospective study of women undergoing ovarian stimulation will provide more insights as to possible aetiological roles; however the presence of persistent ovarian enlargement warrants further investigation to rule out a tumour. Ovarian size should be monitored by ultrasound during and after treatment especially if any abnormality is noted on an initial scan. Other helpful diagnostic tools include transvaginal colour flow imaging (Weiner *et al.* 1992; Kawai *et al.* 1992), serum inhibin levels (Lappohn *et al.* 1989) and ovarian biopsy. In the long term, setting up national registries of patients who have sought fertility evaluation and/or those who were administered ovarian stimulants, will go a long way towards clarifying present clinical suspicions. Patients should be fully informed of the present state of research on this and other complications that may affect their long-term welfare, before obtaining their written consent for treatment.

**Infection**

The incidence of pelvic infection following IUI has been estimated to lie within the range of 0.01–0.20% (Horvath *et al.* 1989; Dodson & Haney 1991; Sacks & Simon 1991; Ombelet *et al.* 1995a). This should not be taken to mean that the incidence of bacterial contamination of the uterine and peritoneal cavities is not higher than this. In fact, Stone and colleagues (1986) demonstrated bacteria in the peritoneal fluid of five out of nine patients who had IUI with prepared sperm suspension. Possible sources of these bacteria include the prepared sperm suspension, using a non-sterile technique for sperm preparation or insemination, or contaminating the tip of the insemination catheter with vaginal organisms before passing it through the cervical canal and into the uterine cavity. The procedure of IUI may also reactivate a chronic pelvic infection.

Semen is not sterile and a recent study identified *Ureaplasma urealyticum, Gardnerella vaginalis, Lactobacillus sp., Staphylococcus epidermidis, Staphylococcus aureus, Staphylococcus capitis, Proteus mirabilis* and *Streptococcus milleri* in semen produced by a group of infertile patients (Boucher *et al.* 1995). Other studies (references in Sacks & Simon 1991) have demonstrated transmission of *Neisseria gonorrhoeae, Streptococcus sp., Trichomonas vaginalis, Ureaplasma urealyticum*, hepatitis B virus, herpes virus

Table 13.8. *Organisms that can be found in semen*

| | |
|---|---|
| *Bacteria, fungi and related organisms* | |
| Candida albicans | Proteus mirabilis |
| Chlamydia trachomatis | Staphylococcus aureus |
| Escherichia coli | Staphylococcus capitis |
| Gardnerella vaginalis | Staphylococcus epidermidis |
| Lactobacillus sp. | Streptococcus milleri |
| Mycobacterium tuberculosis | Streptococcus faecalis |
| Mycoplasma hominis | Trichomonas vaginalis |
| Neisseria gonorrhoea | Ureaplasma urealyticum |
| *Viruses* | |
| Human immunodeficiency virus | |
| Human T cell lymphotrophic virus type 1 | |
| Hepatitis B virus | |
| Hepatitis C virus | |
| Herpes virus | |
| Cytomegalovirus | |
| Human papilloma virus | |

and human immunodeficiency virus through intracervical or intravaginal insemination with unscreened donor semen. Resident bacterial flora of the urethra, glans penis and the hands can also contaminate the ejaculate produced by masturbation. Another source of contamination is the airborne bacteria in the semen collection room. Use of unsterile containers for collection of the ejaculate or during sperm preparation in the laboratory may introduce bacteria into the sample. A list of seminal pathogens can be found in Table 13.8 (Sacks & Simon 1991; Mortimer 1994a; Boucher *et al.* 1995).

Although sperm preparation methods that involve sperm migration or centrifugation through density gradient media such as Percoll (Pharmacia LKB Biotechnology, Uppsala, Sweden) remove virtually all bacteria contained in the semen sample (Mortimer 1994b) this is not invariable; the inseminated sample can still contain bacteria. The fact that pelvic inflammatory disease is most common in sexually active females is ample evidence of the ability of vaginally deposited seminal bacteria to ascend the female genital tract and reach the peritoneal cavity following sexual intercourse. One way this is achieved is by bacteria becoming attached to motile sperms which carry them through the cervical canal, uterine cavity and fallopian tubes. The question is, why is pelvic infection not more common following IUI or normal intercourse? The answer probably lies in the existence of efficient host defence mechanisms

Table 13.9. *Reduction of bacterial contamination of semen during collection*

1. Void urine.
2. Wash hands, forearms and genital area with bactericidal and antifungal soap.
3. Make sure glans penis is washed with foreskin drawn back.
4. Rinse carefully (with sterile water).
5. Dry with sterile gauze or towel.
6. Keep hands away from external urethral meatus during masturbation.
7. Open container just before ejaculation.
8. Avoid touching inner surface of container with penis or hand.

*Notes:*
Adapted from Boucher *et al.* (1995)

which guarantee clearance of micro-organisms that breach the anatomical and physiological barrier placed by the cervix and its secretions. Infection then can only occur where there is a breakdown of these defence mechanisms or the virulence of the organism overwhelms the body's defences.

Another problem in this issue of pelvic infection following artificial insemination, is that diagnosis of infection in most studies is by means of clinical features rather than through bacteriological examination of specimens obtained from the upper genital tract or pelvic cavity. This obviously means that many of the so-called infective episodes may in actual fact be some other reactive phenomenon such as a clinically apparent immunological response to inseminated antigenic proteins. None of the studies that was reviewed by Sacks and Simon (1991) employed bacteriological methods to document the clinical impression of pelvic infection.

Adoption of certain measures will guarantee maintenance of the very low incidence of pelvic infection in females who have IUI. Boucher *et al.* (1995) discussed a number of such measures which they proved in their study decreases bacterial contamination of the sample produced by masturbation (Table 13.9). These instructions are given verbally to the patient before masturbation and this affords him the opportunity of clarifying any misconceptions or seeking more information. The utility of these verbal instructions was subsequently confirmed when it was shown that there was a significant reduction of bacterial contamination of the sample in this group of men as compared to another group who did not receive any verbal instruction apart from being asked to void urine before going into the room where they were to read the printed instructions pasted on the wall. There is a risk that some men may find this approach off putting but this was not shown to be a problem as semen volume was the same in both groups of men studied (Boucher et al. 1995) indicating similar sexual arousal during masturbation. It may however not be practicable for a man to interrupt the act of masturbation to unscrew and remove the cap of the container just prior to ejaculation. A compromise may be for the cap to be unscrewed fully but left lying loosely on top of the container before commencing masturbation. It then becomes easier lifting up this cap, keeping it on the table top and then picking up the container which is used for collecting the ejaculate. Using a wide mouth container (6 cm in diameter instead of 4 cm) makes it easier to avoid touching the inner aspect of the container with the hand or penis.

The benefit of prophylactic antibiotic administration to the patient at the time of IUI or the addition of antibiotics such as penicillin and streptomycin to the culture medium that is used for sperm preparation and insemination has not been determined. This may not be an easy exercise given the very low incidence of pelvic infection after IUI. If the principles utilised elsewhere in medicine are invoked here, no antibiotic prophylaxis should be administered. Instead the patient's clinical state is followed up closely after IUI; she is told to report to the unit if she feels unwell in any way. Careful evaluation at that time, which should incorporate microbiological techniques, will reveal those with pelvic infection who can then be treated promptly and effectively with the indicated antibiotics. Screening of sperm donors and quarantine of semen to enable re-testing of the donors has resulted in their becoming a low risk group for transmitting infection to female donor sperm recipients. Any female who is deemed at risk of pelvic infection by virtue of a significant previous medical history should probably not have IUI in the first place although some may argue for IUI under appropriate prophylactic antibiotic cover. The latter option goes against the ethos of IUI, i.e. a minimally invasive, low cost, less complicated assisted conception treatment alternative to IVF and its variants.

### Non-infective salpingitis

Percoll (Pharmacia LKB Biotechnology, Uppsala, Sweden) is made of silica particles that are coated with polyvinyl pyrrolidone, and silica is a well-known tissue irritant. Concern has been expressed about the use of Percoll during sperm preparation for IUI (Mortimer 1994b) since theoretically, it can cause chemical salpingitis but there does not appear to have been any report of this in the literature so far. The options would be to avoid Percoll and use other buoyant density gradient media such as Ficoll (Pharmacia LKB Biotechnology, Uppsala, Sweden) or Nycondenz (Nyegaard, Oslo, Norway), or to adopt a very careful approach to ensure removal of as much Percoll as possible, during the washing steps following initial centrifugation of the semen sample through Percoll. Similar considerations probably apply to PureSperm (NidaCon Laboratories AB, Gothenburg, Sweden) and ISolate (Irvine Scientific, Santa Ana, USA) which are now being used instead of Percoll for sperm preparation during human assisted conception treatment.

### Allergic reactions

Allergic reactions to bovine serum albumin (Sonenthal *et al.* 1991) and penicillin (Smith *et al.* 1992) have been reported following IUI of prepared sperm suspended in culture media containing these compounds. Severe uterine contractions, dyspnoea, chest tightness, pruritus and urticaria began within 5 minutes of IUI in one patient (Sonenthal *et al.* 1991) while it took 6 hours for symptoms of urticaria on the limbs and trunk, and oedema of the hands and eyelids to appear in the other patient (Smith *et al.* 1992). The patient who was allergic to bovine serum albumin did not have a history of such a problem but she suffered from asthma and was known to be allergic to penicillin and phenytoin while the woman who reacted to penicillin had a positive history of penicillin allergy. Subsequent skin testing confirmed the existence of sensitisation in the two patients. The occurrence of these reactions is particularly striking given the extremely small amount of the offending agent contained in the inseminated volumes.

Although only a few cases have been reported some others may go unrecognised by the clinician if they are mild, transient and occur after the patient has left the unit. Some cases may not manifest until after many hours have elapsed from the time of insemination (Smith *et al.* 1992) and the patient may not establish the connection between the two events. Because of the very small number of reported cases it is not yet possible to determine the role of insemination, with media containing allergenic substances, as the primary sensitisation event. This notwithstanding, repeated cycles of insemination are likely to boost the level of relevant immunoglobulins in those who are already sensitised thereby increasing the severity of the reaction.

A complete history of allergies, especially to antibiotics and other drugs or animal products, should be sought in all patients as part of the general workup during infertility consultations, especially before assisted conception treatment. Antibiotics should be omitted from culture media used for sperm preparation for insemination in individuals with suggestive previous histories which could include that of atopic illness such as eczema and asthma. The use of heat-inactivated human serum albumin as the protein source for culture media may remove the problem of sensitisation by albumin of animal origin.

An alternative would be for the patient's serum to be used in preparing the culture medium. The serum should be heat treated by maintaining the sample at 60 °C for 10 hours to destroy any pathogens which it may contain. This is important for the prevention of cross infection of other samples being handled at the same time and for the protection of staff. A protective effect from antibiotics contained in culture media on post-insemination pelvic infection has not been demonstrated convincingly, so they should be avoided when making culture medium that will come into intimate contact with the patient. This is because there will always be the potential danger of a severe life threatening anaphylactic reaction to the penicillin contained in the insemination medium as up to 10% of the population may have this allergy.

**Antisperm antibodies**

IUI delivers a relatively large antigenic load of sperm to the upper female genital tract and, perhaps, the peritoneal cavity, so it is theoretically possible for this procedure to lead to the generation of antisperm antibodies in women. The fact that this has not been reported as a common occurrence following IUI suggests that modulatory factors are involved and they determine which females will become sensitised. Kremer (1979) concluded in his study that IUI did not provoke antisperm antibody formation in non-sensitised females, but in those who already had moderately high serum antisperm antibody titres, IUI increased the titre further. Interestingly, a patient who experienced increasing antibody titres during the course of repeated cycles of IUI became pregnant at the fourth attempt. This illustrates the often poor correlation of the presence and titre of serum antisperm antibodies with infertility. Friedman *et al.* (1991) in their study of 51 infertile women who had a mean of four cycles of IUI found 9.8% (five patients) and 6.1% (three patients) to have developed serum and cervical mucus antisperm antibodies, respectively.

Paradoxically, no antisperm antibodies were detectable after IUI in three women who previously had antibodies. Furthermore, none of the women with cervical mucus or serum based antisperm antibodies had demonstrated further increases in antibody titres after IUI. Finally, there was no correlation between the number of IUI cycles performed in each case and development of antisperm antibodies (Friedman *et al.* 1991). Further study is needed here and the first step should be to identify protective immunological mechanisms that prevent sensitisation of most females to sperm antigens despite their leading very active sexual lives. It could be that those who go on to develop antisperm antibodies have a breakdown or poor functioning of such protective mechanisms.

## Miscarriage

It is believed that the miscarriage rate is high in pregnancies conceived as a result of assisted conception treatment and rates of between 20 and 30% have been quoted in the literature (Schenker & Ezra 1994). The reason for this is not known with certainty but may be related to the relatively older age of the woman presenting for assisted conception treatment. An older age is associated with an increased incidence of chromosomal abnormalities in the oocyte, and hence the resulting conceptus (Schenker & Ezra 1994). The possibility exists that the greater early pregnancy wastage, common in multiple pregnancies ordinarily, reflect on the miscarriage rate figures following assisted conception treatment as there is a higher incidence of multiple pregnancies in the latter situation. The exact background miscarriage rate in the general population is unknown. Most workers would agree that the apparently high rate found in pregnancies after assisted conception treatment can be partly explained by the greater intensity of monitoring of these women. It is likely that many cases of early pregnancy loss are not diagnosed in the general population and would not be reflected in epidemiological data. Miscarriage rates following IUI seem to lie within the same range found after IVF and its variants (Ombelet *et al.* 1995b).

## Ectopic pregnancy

The incidence of ectopic pregnancy shows a marked regional variation in spontaneously conceived pregnancies, being higher in urban areas than in rural communities. The main reason for this difference is the proportionately higher prevalence of pelvic inflammatory disease and its sequelae in urban centres. There is well-documented evidence to show that ectopic pregnancies are more common in women who have a history of pelvic infection. This effect of pelvic disease on ectopic pregnancy rates also manifests after assisted conception treatment since many women who have this treatment do so as a result of infertility resulting from tubal or peritubal lesions (Schenker & Ezra 1994). The incidence of ectopic pregnancy in these women is between 3 and 5.5% (Schenker & Ezra 1994) and does not seem to be different after IUI as compared to other assisted conception treatments (Ombelet *et al.* 1995b). Further studies are needed to clarify these figures as any patient having IUI is not expected to have tubal disease if case selection is properly carried out in any centre. The ectopic pregnancy rate should therefore be lower after IUI than that obtaining in IVF and related treatments where tubal disease is not a contraindication. Normal findings at hysterosalpingography and laparoscopy with chromotubation do not exclude mucosal tubal pathology which can also arrest the transit of the embryo along the tube thereby leading to ectopic pregnancy.

Visualisation of an intrauterine gestation is usually regarded as strong evidence to support the exclusion of an ectopic pregnancy in natural conceptions. This is because the risk of a coexisting ectopic pregnancy is quite small, being quoted at between 1 in 5000 to 1 in 15000 pregnancies. This figure is a function of the ectopic and multiple pregnancy rates in that particular community. It is then logical that the incidence of heterotopic pregnancies (i.e. coexisting intrauterine and ectopic pregnancies) should be higher in assisted conception treatment cycles. Rates of between 1 in 83 and 1 in 200 have been quoted for all pregnancies resulting from assisted conception treatments (Schenker & Ezra 1994) but specific figures for IUI are needed.

Ectopic pregnancy is a potentially life-threatening condition which further jeopardises the fertility potential of the patient; however, with the introduction of better diagnostic aids the number of cases detected prior to tubal rupture and bleeding into the peritoneal cavity has gradually increased. Consequently, minimally invasive alternatives to traditional surgical treatments were developed thereby permitting a decrease in post-operative morbidity and an increased preservation of reproductive function. A previous history of ectopic pregnancy is an indication for a cautious approach towards the management of future conceptions. A careful transvaginal ultrasound evaluation of the uterus, fallopian tubes and pelvic cavity is required from 5 weeks of gestation onwards, to exclude a recurrence which is not unusual. This becomes more important in pregnancies that result from assisted conception treatments; however it is not appropriate to manage a patient having such a previous medical history with IUI despite tubal patency being established. This is because these patients are already predisposed to having ectopic pregnancies and may have coexisting intratubal lesions that will impede the passage of the early embryo on its way to implanting in the uterine cavity. Ectopic pregnancy has been extensively dealt with in the book by Stabile (1996).

## Conclusion

The above account has attempted to present useful information for the prevention and treatment of the common complications met with during or as a result of IUI. A few other problems deserve mention although they are less commonly encountered. Some difficulty may be experienced with cannulation of the cervical canal during IUI and this is more likely in those with stenosed cervices or sharply anteverted or retroverted uteri. There is a broad range of available insemination catheters which with skill and patience could be used safely and atraumatically to gain access to the uterine cavity for insemination. Occasional bleeding may occur afterwards from trauma to the epithelium of the cervical canal or from the point of application of vulsellum forceps in difficult cases. Intraperitoneal insemination is an option in such cases. Vasovagal symptoms may rarely occur on cervical instrumentation especially in nulliparous patients. Uterine cramps occur in a minority of patients despite the use of washed sperm samples for IUI. Poor response to ovarian stimulation and insemination with the wrong sperm sample are other complications with the latter being a complete disaster which should be avoidable if a system of checks and counterchecks is put in place for the confirmation of the identity of sperm suspensions before insemination.

**References**

Amso N. (1995) Ovarian hyperstimulation syndrome: prevention and management. In: *Advances in Reproductive Endocrinology, vol. 7: Assisted Reproduction; Progress in Research and Practice*. (R. W. Shaw, ed.), Parthenon Publishing Group, Carnforth, pp. 93–102.

Amso N. N., Shaw R. W., Ahuja K. K. & Morris N. (1991) Prevention of ovarian hyperstimulation syndrome. *Fertility and Sterility* **55**, 220 (letter).

Asch R. H., Ivery E., Goldsman M., Frederick J. L., Stone S. C. & Balmaceda J. P. (1993) The use of intravenous albumin in patients at high risk for severe ovarian hyperstimulation syndrome. *Fertility and Sterility* **8**, 1015–1020.

Balasch J. & Barri P. N. (1993) Follicular stimulation and ovarian cancer? *Human Reproduction* **8**, 990–996.

BNF (1992) *British National Formulary*. No. 24 (September 1992).

Boucher P., Lejeune H., Pinatel C. & Gille Y. (1995) Spermoculture: improvement of the bacteriological quality of samples by direct verbal counseling before semen collection. *Fertility and Sterility* **64**, 657–660.

Brinsden P. R., Wada I., Tan S. L., Balen A. & Jacobs H. S. (1995) Diagnosis, prevention and management of ovarian hyperstimulation syndrome. *British Journal of Obstetrics and Gynaecology* **102**, 767–772.

Cohen J., Forman R., Harlap S., Johannison E., Lunenfeld B., de Mouzon J., Pepperell R., Tarlatzis B. & Templeton A. (1993) IFFS expert group report on the Whittemore study related to the risk of ovarian cancer associated with the use of infertility agents. *Human Reproduction* **8**, 996–999.

Dodson W. C. & Haney A. F. (1991) Controlled ovarian hyperstimulation and intrauterine insemination for treatment of infertility. *Fertility and Sterility* **55**, 457–467.

Fishel S. & Jackson P. (1989) Follicular stimulation for high tech pregnancies: are we playing it safe? *British Medical Journal* **299**, 309–311.

Forman R. G., Frydman R. & Egan D. (1990) Severe ovarian hyperstimulation syndrome using agonists of gonadotrophin releasing hormone for in vitro fertilisation: a European series and a proposal for prevention. *Fertility and Sterility* **53**, 502–509.

Friedman A. J., Juneau-Norcross M. & Sedensky B. (1991) Antisperm antibody production following intrauterine insemination. *Human Reproduction* **6**, 1125–1128.

Friedman A. J., Juneau-Norcross M., Sedensky B., Andrews N., Dorfman J. & Cramer D. W. (1992) Life-table analysis of intrauterine insemination pregnancy rates for couples with cervical factor, male factor and idiopathic infertility. *Fertility and Sterility* **55**, 1005–1007.

Golan A., Ron-El R., Herman A., Soffer Y., Weinraub Z. & Caspi E. (1989) Ovarian hyperstimulation syndrome: an update review. *Obstetrical and Gynecological Survey* **44**, 430–440.

Gonen Y., Balakier H., Powell W. & Casper R. F. (1990) Use of gonadotrophin-releasing hormone agonist to trigger follicular maturation for in vitro fertilisation. *Journal of Clinical Endocrinology and Metabolism* **71**, 918–922.

Harris R., Whittemore A. S., Intyre J., the Collaborative Ovarian Cancer Group (1992) Characteristics relating to ovarian cancer risk: collaborative analysis of 12 US case-control studies. 3. Epithelial tumors of low malignant potential in white women. *American Journal of Epidemiology* **136**, 1204–1211.

Horn-Ross P. L., Whittemore A. S., Intyre J., the Collaborative Ovarian Cancer Group (1992) Characteristics relating to ovarian cancer risk: collaborative analysis of 12 US case-control studies. 4. Non-epithelial cancers among adults. *Epidemiology* **3**, 490–495.

Horvath P. M., Bohrer M., Shelden R. M. & Kemmann E. (1989) The relationship of sperm parameters to cycle fecundity in superovulated women undergoing intra-uterine insemination. *Fertility and Sterility* **52**, 288–294.

Kawai M., Kano T., Kikkawa F., Maeda O., Oguchi H. & Tomoda Y. (1992) Transvaginal doppler ultrasound with color flow imaging in the diagnosis of ovarian cancer. *Obstetrics and Gynecology* **79**, 163–167.

Kremer J. (1979) A new technique for intrauterine insemination. *International Journal of Fertility* **24**, 53–56.

Lappohn R. E., Burger H. G., Bouma J., Bangah M., Krans M. & De Bruijn H. W. A. (1989) Inhibin as a marker for granulosa-cell tumors. *New England Journal of Medicine* **321**, 790–793.

Lipitz S., Ben-Rafael Z., Bider D., Shalev J. & Mashiach S. (1991) Quintuplet pregnancy and third degree ovarian hyperstimulation despite witholding human chorionic gonadotrophin. *Human Reproduction* **6**, 1478–1479.

Mashiach S., Bider D., Moran O., Goldenberg M. & Ben-Rafael Z. (1990) Adnexal torsion of hyperstimulated ovaries in pregnancies after gonadotrophin therapy. *Fertility and Sterility* **53**, 76–80.

Mortimer D. (1994a) Semen microbiology and virology. In: *Practical Laboratory Andrology*. Oxford University Press, Oxford, pp. 127–133.

Mortimer D. (1994b) Sperm washing. In: *Practical Laboratory Andrology*. Oxford University Press, Oxford, pp. 267–286.

Ombelet W., Cox A., Jansen M., Vandeput H. & Bosmans E. (1995a) Artificial insemination (AIH). Artificial insemination 2: using the husband's sperm. In: *Diagnosis and Therapy of Male Factor in Assisted Reproduction*. (A. A. Acosta, T. F. Kruger, eds), The Parthenon Publishing Group, Carnforth, pp. 397–410.

Ombelet W., Puttemans P. & Bosmans E. (1995b) Intrauterine insemination: a first-step procedure in the algorithm of male subfertility treatment. *Human Reproduction* **10** (supplement), 90–102.

Rabau E., Serr D. M., David A., Mashiach S. & Lunenfeld B. (1967) Human menopausal gonadotrophins for anovulation and sterility. *American Journal of Obstetrics and Gynecology* **98**, 92–98.

Rizk B. (1992) Ovarian hyperstimulation syndrome. In: *A Textbook of In Vitro*

*Fertilization and Assisted Reproduction.* (P. R. Brinsden, P. A. Rainsbury, eds), The Parthenon Publishing Group, Carnforth, pp. 369–383.

Rossing M. A., Daling J. R., Weiss N. S., Moore D. E. & Self S. G. (1994) Ovarian tumors in a cohort of infertile women. *New England Journal of Medicine* **331**, 771–776.

Sacks P. C. & Simon J. A. (1991) Infectious complications of intrauterine insemination: a case report and literature review. *International Journal of Fertility* **36**, 331–339.

Schenker J. G. & Ezra Y. (1994) Complications of assisted reproductive techniques. *Fertility and Sterility* **61**, 411–422.

Schenker J. G. & Weinstein D. (1978) Ovarian hyperstimulation syndrome: a current survey. *Fertility and Sterility* **30**, 255–268.

Shahata M., Yang D., Al-Natsha S. D. & Al-Shawaf T. (1994) Intravenous albumin and severe ovarian hyperstimulation. *Human Reproduction* **9**, 2186.

Shoham Z., Weissman A., Barash A., Borenstein R., Schachter M. & Insler V. (1994) Intravenous albumin for the prevention of severe ovarian hyperstimulation syndrome in an in vitro fertilisation programme: a prospective randomised, placebo-controlled study. *Fertility and Sterility* **62**, 137–142.

Shushan A., Paltiel O., Iscovich J., Elchalal U., Peretz T. & Schenker J. G. (1996) Human menopausal gonadotropin and the risk of epithelial ovarian cancer. *Fertility and Sterility* **65**, 13–18.

Smith Y. R., Hurd W. W., Menge A. C., Sanders G. M., Ansbacher R. & Randolph J. F. (1992) Allergic reactions to penicillin during in vitro fertilization and intrauterine insemination. *Fertility and Sterility* **58**, 847–849.

Sonenthal K. R., McKnight T., Shaughnessy M. A., Grammer L. C. & Jeyendran R. S. (1991) Anaphylaxis during intrauterine insemination secondary to bovine serum albumin. *Fertility and Sterility* **56**, 1188–1191.

Stone S. C., de la Marza L. M. & Peterson E. M. (1986) Recovery of microorganisms from the pelvic cavity after intracervical or intrauterine artificial insemination. *Fertility and Sterility* **46**, 61–65.

Stabile I. (1996) *Ectopic Pregnancy: Diagnosis and Management.* Cambridge University Press, Cambridge.

Tan S. L. (1994) Luteinizing hormone-releasing hormone agonists for ovarian stimulation in assisted reproduction. *Current Opinion in Obstetrics and Gynecology* **6**, 166–172.

Taubert H.-D. & Kuhl H. (1994) Steroids and steroid-like compounds. In: *Infertility: Male and Female.* (V. Insler, B. Lunenfeld, eds), second. edition, Churchill Livingstone, Edinburgh, pp. 435–480.

Tsirigotis M. & Craft I. (1994) Ovarian hyperstimulation syndrome (OHSS): how much do we really know about it? *European Journal of Obstetrics and Gynecology and Reproductive Biology* **55**, 151–155.

Venn A., Watson L., Lumley J., Giles G., King C. & Healy D. (1995) Breast and ovarian cancer incidence after infertility and in vitro fertilisation. *Lancet* **346**, 995–1000.

Wada I., Macnamee M. & Brinsden P. (1993a) Prevention and treatment of ovarian hyperstimulation. *Human Reproduction* **8**, 2245–2247 (letter).

Wada I., Matson P. L., Troup S. A., Hughes S. M., Buck P. & Lieberman B. A. (1992) Outcome of treatment subsequent to the elective cryopreservation of all embryos from women at risk of the ovarian hyperstimulation syndrome. *Human Reproduction* **7**, 962–966.

Wada I., Matson P. L., Troup S. A., Morroll D., Hunt L. & Lieberman B. A. (1993b) Does elective cryopreservation of all embryos from women at risk of ovarian hyperstimulation syndrome reduce the incidence of the condition? *British Journal of Obstetrics and Gynaecology* **100**, 265–269.

Waterstone J., Bennett S., Ribeiro R., Curson R. & Parsons J. (1991) Prevention and management of ovarian hyperstimulation syndrome. *Lancet* **338**, 1536–1537.

Weiner Z., Thaler I., Beck D., Rottem S., Deutsch M. & Brandes J. M. (1992) Differentiating malignant from benign ovarian tumors with transvaginal color flow imaging. *Obstetrics and Gynecology* **79**, 159–162.

Whittemore A. S. (1993) Fertility drugs and the risk of ovarian cancer. *Human Reproduction* **8**, 999–1000.

Whittemore A. S., Harris R., Intyre J., the Collaborative Ovarian Cancer Group (1992) Characteristics relating to ovarian cancer risk: collaborative analysis of twelve US case-control studies. 2. invasive epithelial ovarian cancer in white women. *American Journal of Epidemiology* **136**, 1184–1203.

Willemsen W., Kruitwagen R., Bastiaans B., Hanselaar T. & Rolland R. (1993) Ovarian stimulation and granulosa-cell tumour. *Lancet* **341**, 986–988.

# 14

## Concluding remarks: thoughts on the management of infertility

GODWIN I. MENIRU

The true incidence of infertility is difficult to ascertain but evidence so far indicates that it is common with rates lying in the range of 10–30%. Fertility presents a spectrum of varying propensity for natural conception. Some couples are able to establish pregnancies with ease while others may experience differing degrees of difficulty before being successful but individuals whose fertility potential lies at the opposite end of the spectrum never do so because they are sterile. Fertility in a couple is a function of time as well as being determined by the fertility of each partner. One partner's fertility potential may compensate for a reduction of the other's fertility but a different outcome may be experienced if the fertility of both partners is reduced or one of them is sterile.

It is not surprising that infertility is so common, as conception in the human is an inefficient process. The human female does not exhibit any features that will alert the male to the fact that she is about to ovulate. Sexual intercourse does not trigger off ovulation unlike some other mammalian species and fertilisation of an ovulated oocyte depends on a chance meeting with sperms in the fallopian tubes. Although several million sperms are contained in the ejaculate only a very small proportion successfully escape the hostile conditions of the vagina by entering the cervical canal. A few hundreds, or at most a few thousands, are found at the site of fertilisation in the fallopian tubes. The oocyte usually allows only one sperm to bind with and penetrate the oolemma. There are regional variations in the distribution of different causes of infertility and clinic-based figures will be biased towards greater representation of those infertility factors in which clinical and scientific staff have special interests and expertise. Some causes, such as tubal damage from pelvic infection, are related to social influences but many others are not. This is probably why infertility will continue to affect a significant proportion of the populace notwithstanding future medical and scientific advances. An increasing knowledge of the determinants and pathophysiology of fertility problems will however improve the efficacy of treatment modalities.

The time of presentation at the clinic varies depending on individual circumstances although regional and ethnic factors may affect this too. Some couples may present early, just after a few months of trying while others present after several years, by which time natural reproductive function could already be waning. Each case has to be treated on its own merits but reassurance and support of couples who present early to the clinic can only be realistically performed after a full evaluation of the couple, and this should not be regarded as premature intervention. If no sterilising abnormality is discovered the couple can then be reassured and offered conservative measures aimed at optimising their chances of natural conception. Follow-up clinic appointments are provided so as to make sure they are not forgotten. If, however, a pathology that requires treatment is uncovered, the couple would then have benefited from an early diagnosis and referral for treatment.

Another dimension to the problem of infertility is seen following presentation at the primary care gynaecological clinic. A large proportion of couples spend many years at these clinics, making repeated hospital visits, having an endless number of investigations and being administered ineffective treatment. A major advance in fertility management will occur when clinicians become more efficient in their evaluation of infertile couples and recognise the importance of time dependent changes in both natural reproductive function and response to assisted conception treatment. Furthermore, generalist specialists should learn how to relinquish control of patients to colleagues who have special interests and skills in the management of infertility. This naturally leads to the question of who is best suited to manage infertile patients. Is it the family practitioner, generalist gynaecologist or reproductive medicine subspecialist? The simple answer is that anyone can do so, provided he or she is skilled and well informed on the current perspectives of fertility management, and does not constitute an impediment to the speedy and effective treatment of these patients. The three groups of physicians actually have well defined roles which if carried out properly will make managing infertile patients more efficient and cost-effective.

A pragmatic approach should be adopted once a couple is referred with a complaint of difficulty in achieving pregnancy. A complete medical history is obtained and each partner is examined carefully, followed by relevant investigations which can often be completed within the time frame of one menstrual cycle (Figure 14.1). Investigations can be commenced at any point in the menstrual cycle. Additional tests are performed when indicated. Relevant texts should be consulted for further information on these investigations. At the end

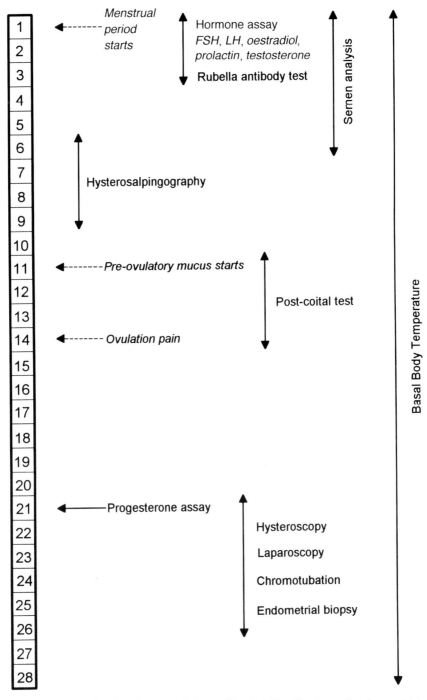

Figure 14.1. A plan for the completion of basic infertility investigations within one menstrual cycle.

of this evaluation it will often be possible to identify a broad range of problems including ovulatory dysfunction, tubal blockage, endometriosis, tubo-ovarian lesions and abnormal sperm parameters. The aetiological basis of infertility in a couple is often multifactorial and both partners must have the standard investigations notwithstanding the fact that one partner might already have been shown to have an infertility-associated problem. No abnormaility, however, will be found in a significant proportion of couples and these are said to have unexplained infertility. The incidence of this diagnosis depends to a large extent on how extensive the infertility investigation is but care should be taken to avoid exposing the couple to an unnecessary battery of tests many of which may have poor predictive values. Distinction should always be made between tests that are still under evaluation and those that have been shown to contribute significantly to the clinical management of couples. The opportunity afforded by this contact with medical facilities should be properly utilised to ensure that preventive medical care of the couple is up to date. Thus the woman should have breast examination, cervical smears and a rubella immune status check while the man is taught how to examine his testes for new swellings. Their blood pressure and urine samples are checked together with their history of other immunisations, especially for polio and tetanus. Finally, an enquiry into lifestyle factors such as smoking, diet and exercise is carried out.

If an infertility-associated problem is identified and it is within the competence of the clinician to treat, proper treatment should then be given and the couple monitored closely to determine the success or otherwise of the treatment. The couple should be referred to a subspecialist for the management of more complex problems. The treatment of any particular problem should be put in its correct perspective by comparing expected gains from the treatment with temporary exacerbation of the infertile state. Medical treatment of endometriosis, for example, often involves suppression of ovarian activity for periods of up to 6 months and above, thereby extending the period of infertility further. This is compounded by the fact that restoration of normal fertility is not invariable after such treatments. Treatment of endometriosis may not be appropriate in some cases such as the older woman with several years of infertility and asymptomatic mild disease. These women should be considered for assisted conception treatment without delay. For patients in whom no obvious cause for the infertility is found, further management options will depend on the female patient's age, period of infertility and the wishes of the couple. At one extreme, simple reassurance and reproductive health education may be all that is needed while at the other end, immediate referral for assisted conception treatment will be required. It is quite clear that a significant proportion of infertile patients with non-sterilising defects do become pregnant spontaneously. In fact it is estimated that only 3–4% of women will remain sterile at the end of their reproductive lives. There is no doubt that 'time heals infertility' but there are also situations in which it is quite inappropriate continuing to wait for the spontaneous resolution of infertility in a couple.

Infertile patients had severely limited treatment options up to 30 years ago but this has changed following the first birth, in 1978, of an infant conceived extracorporally. The assisted reproduction technologies have now enabled a continually increasing number of couples to achieve pregnancies and these techniques have become established as clinical treatment options for infertility. In vitro fertilisation (IVF) and its variants are invasive and expensive, and success is not guaranteed in any particular cycle of treatment. Re-discovery of intrauterine insemination (IUI), which in the current form involves sperm preparation and insemination in a superovulated cycle, means that less invasive and cheaper options are now available for certain classes of patients. IUI has been shown to be effective in many studies but other reports show poor results and it is not immediately apparent why these widely fluctuating pregnancy rates continue to be reported. The most likely explanation is that there is a myriad of variables which can affect outcome of IUI and are rarely represented proportionately in the different reports (Figure 14.2). Furthermore, many of these studies are retrospective, involve relatively small patient numbers and do not provide enough information to make their comparison or meta-analysis useful.

One of the best ways of obtaining meaningful information on IUI that will enable definite conclusions on its efficacy would be to organise a collaborative prospective multicentre study which would aim at acquiring data on many thousand cycles of treatment. By doing so it will become possible to examine the contribution of each factor to success at IUI. Additionally, the large database will allow the use of relevant statistics to determine the impact of various confounding variables on results of IUI. This writer does not feel that the proposed study should be prescriptive because it is an exploratory exercise and participation by as many units as possible will help achieve the goal of establishing such a large database. Each participating centre will be allowed to continue carrying out IUI as it normally does but all requested information on each cycle entered into the study must be submitted. The data will reflect on the variables shown in Figure 14.2 and will be in currently accepted formats. Diagnosis of the cause of infertility, for example, can only be accepted if a certain number of stated investigations were carried out. Thus any patient who did not have laparoscopy and chromotubation cannot be deemed to be free of tubal, peritubal or pelvic disease. This writer will welcome comments on the design of this study from the readers.

Infertility evokes complex psychological responses in individuals and this may be worsened by the attitude of friends, relatives and workplace companions. Society has generally been unsupportive of infertile patients and this is highlighted by the lack of incorporation of assisted conception treatments within the framework of traditional health care entitlement in most countries. This is despite the fact that these couples are highly productive members of the society who contribute to all forms of medical care insurance schemes, be they governmental or privately owned. Relying on these couples to force a change in the attitude of the society at large may not be fruitful as they are usually not militant, unlike some other groups that are discriminated against. They tend to suffer their infertility in silence and continued callous pronouncements, by the fertile majority, such as 'infertility is not a disease', wound them deeply. It is probably only time and education of the populace that will reverse this state of affairs but public spirited individuals and organisations have a role in accelerating the change.

Psychological issues in infertility are complex and have been dealt with in Chapter 4 which should be read in conjunction with other specialist texts. There is a need for counselling support before, during and after treatment, whether successful or not. Infertility tends to expose unresolved psychological problems in the partners of a couple or deficits in the relationship itself and these may worsen following continued infertility or repeated treatment failure. Counselling therefore has to take cognisance of these and other factors and provide couples with non-dysfunctional coping mechanisms. Infertility treatment by IUI should not be allowed to potentiate any feelings of inadequacy in especially the male partner because fertility is invariably associated by most people with potency and gender identity. Much remains unknown about the best way to deal with these couples but it is likely to be dependent on individual personalities and preferences. Insemination itself should be conducted in a quiet atmosphere and the female partner should not be overexposed.

Opinions vary as to how to maximise the sense of participation in the male partner. Some units will allow the man to depress the plunger of the insemination syringe but this might be an unnecessary interference with medical routine and introduce variability into the practice. This is a symbolic gesture and other ways can still be found to achieve similar effects while maintaining optimal treatment techniques. One issue that does not appear to have been studied yet is the male partner's preference for the sex of the medical worker who performs the insemination. Lesbians seem to prefer the female sex but men may also prefer a female to perform the insemination rather than another male carrying out what he (the patient) might feel he has been unsuccessful in achieving

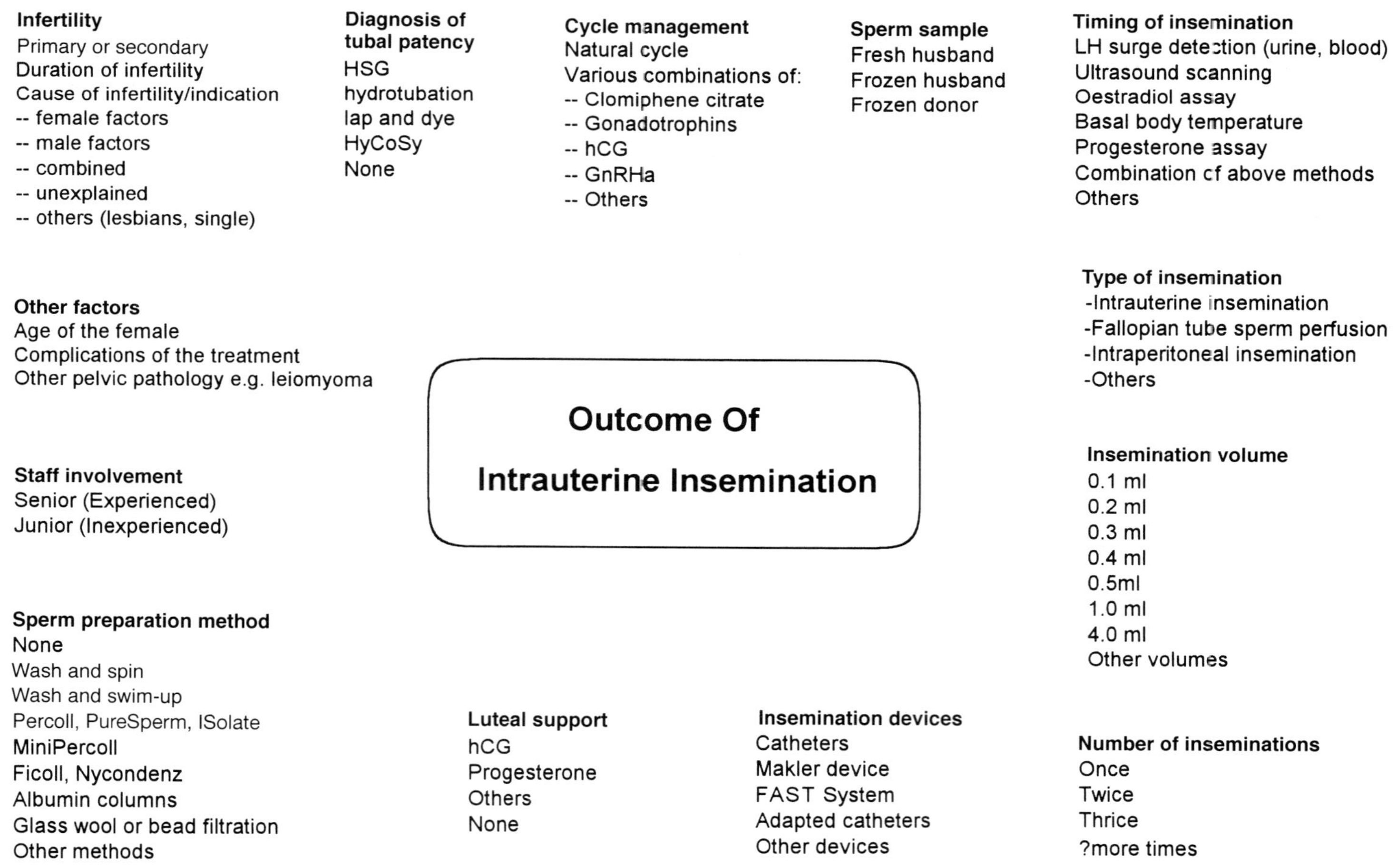

**Infertility**
Primary or secondary
Duration of infertility
Cause of infertility/indication
-- female factors
-- male factors
-- combined
-- unexplained
-- others (lesbians, single)

**Diagnosis of tubal patency**
HSG
hydrotubation
lap and dye
HyCoSy
None

**Cycle management**
Natural cycle
Various combinations of:
-- Clomiphene citrate
-- Gonadotrophins
-- hCG
-- GnRHa
-- Others

**Sperm sample**
Fresh husband
Frozen husband
Frozen donor

**Timing of insemination**
LH surge detection (urine, blood)
Ultrasound scanning
Oestradiol assay
Basal body temperature
Progesterone assay
Combination cf above methods
Others

**Type of insemination**
-Intrauterine insemination
-Fallopian tube sperm perfusion
-Intraperitoneal insemination
-Others

**Other factors**
Age of the female
Complications of the treatment
Other pelvic pathology e.g. leiomyoma

**Staff involvement**
Senior (Experienced)
Junior (Inexperienced)

**Sperm preparation method**
None
Wash and spin
Wash and swim-up
Percoll, PureSperm, ISolate
MiniPercoll
Ficoll, Nycondenz
Albumin columns
Glass wool or bead filtration
Other methods

**Luteal support**
hCG
Progesterone
Others
None

**Insemination devices**
Catheters
Makler device
FAST System
Adapted catheters
Other devices

**Insemination volume**
0.1 ml
0.2 ml
0.3 ml
0.4 ml
0.5ml
1.0 ml
4.0 ml
Other volumes

**Number of inseminations**
Once
Twice
Thrice
?more times

**Outcome Of Intrauterine Insemination**

Figure 14.2. Factors that determine outcome of intrauterine insemination.

naturally. This consideration is even more important in men with erectile or ejaculatory dysfunction.

Other difficulties include mechanisation of sex and masturbation may not be acceptable to some men for religious, cultural, moral or other reasons. This is worsened when the man is asked to produce a sample at the unit rather than in familiar home surroundings and some form of 'performance anxiety' may make this impossible in some cases. This writer has observed that men from certain cultures take a disproportionately long time to produce semen samples by masturbation at the unit. In fact some are unable to do so and have to go back to their lodgings to do this or use an inert silicone rubber non-spermicidal condom (Seminal Collection Condom; Rocket Medical, Watford, UK) to collect the ejaculate during vaginal intercourse. Clinic appointment letters to patient's should mention the requirement for on-site production of semen. Those who would prefer to come to the unit to do so before the day of the first clinic consultation should be encouraged. If any patient has a strong preference for producing the sample at home and bringing it to the unit, this should be allowed. The unit's specimen production room is preferably sited in a quiet part of the complex.

Donor insemination deserves special mention. The decision to use donor semen should not be made without due consideration of all aspects of the case including psychosocial factors. The use of donor semen is not an option for some religious groups although the clinician probably still has a duty to mention at least, the availability of donor semen to individual couples, while at the same time deferring to their wishes. The advent of microassisted fertilisation methods such as intracytoplasmic sperm injection has allowed an increasing number of men to become genetic parents. Donor semen will however be required by some couples due to the presence of hereditary disease in the male and other reasons (see Chapter 3). This is not likely to be an easy step for a man and he needs the support of his spouse and members of the medical team. Chapter 4 deals with other issues to be resolved before donor insemination is undertaken for any couple.

In conclusion, IUI is not a panacea for infertility and should not be regarded as such. There will never be a single treatment for infertility, just a collection of remedies of varying efficacy which are applied to particular couples when indicated. The rightful place of IUI has not yet been determined but all available evidence points to its being a reliable first line assisted conception treatment option. Most pregnancies occur within the first three to four cycles of treatment after which time serious consideration should be given to IVF. This manual was compiled based on this philosophy and it is hoped that the reader will become a more informed practitioner of IUI.

# Index

absentee husbands, 37–8
adhesions, 102, 110
allergy to semen, 34, 226–7
ampoules, 180
anti-neoplastic treatment, 38
antisperm antibodies, 35–7, 227
artificial insemination, 1, 146, 204 see also intrauterine insemination
asthenozoospermia, 30

bleeding, vaginal, 95
buserelin, 62, 89–90

cancer, 220
   anti-neoplastic treatment, 38
   ovarian, 70, 218–22
   uterine, 220
cell membranes, 165
   cryopreservation effects on, 165–7
cervical factor, 32–3
cervical mucus, 32
   hostility, 1, 33
clomiphene citrate, 2, 57–60, 85
   insemination timing and, 81–2
   ovarian hyperstimulation syndrome and, 207
   sole use of, 63–4
   with gonadotrophins, 64–5, 81–2, 86–7
confidentiality, 48–59
congenital absence of the vas deferens, 3
counselling, 46–54, 239
   confidentiality issues, 48–9
   for options, 50
   in vitro fertilization and, 52–3
   insemination and, 50–2
      donor insemination, 51
      male factor infertility and, 51
   multicultural and religious issues, 53
   nurses' role, 161–2
   sperm donors, 191–2
counsellors, 48, 54
cryobanking, 190
   see also donor sperm banking
cryopreservation of semen, 163–85

cellular injury during freeze-thaw cycle, 168–9
cryoprotectants, 164–5, 195–6
   actions of, 168
   addition to semen, 196
   cryoprotective diluents, 176–8
donor semen, 195–202
drug therapy, 39–40
effects on sperm, 182–3
   assessment of, 184–5
   sperm membranes, 165–7
   thawing effects on survival, 183
equipment and materials, 169–74
   glassware washing procedure, 176
indications for, 37–40
   absentee husband, 37–8
   anti-neoplastic treatment, 38
   vasectomy, 38
packaging, 170–2, 179–80, 185, 197
poor semen samples, 178–9
semen collection, 169–70, 174–5
techniques, 180–1, 197–8
   dry ice pelletting, 181
   liquid nitrogen vapour, 180–1
   programmable freezing, 172, 181
   vapour freezing, 172, 181
culture media, 16–18
cyclofenil, 59
cytomegalovirus (CMV), 193–4

density gradient centrifugation, 138–44
   Percoll gradients, 1, 3, 140
   PureSperm, 140–4
donor insemination, 204, 241
   counselling, 50–2
   indications for, 3, 40–1
   matching donor-recipient characteristics, 202–4
donor sperm banking, 190–204
   donor counselling, 191–2
   donor recruitment, 191
   donor screening and selection, 192–4
   filing and coding, 195
   packaging, 197
   semen donation, 195

storage of frozen semen, 198–202 *see also* cryopreservation of semen
dry ice pelletting, 181

Earle's balanced salt solution preparation, 136–7
ectopic pregnancy, 109, 228–9
egg yolk use in cryoprotectant, 164, 195–6
  formulations, 176–7
ejaculation
  dysfunction, 4, 26–8
  retrograde, 24–6
endometriosis, 34–5, 66, 110
  treatment of, 237
  ultrasound diagnosis, 103–4
endometrium, sonographic evaluation of, 118–24

Fallopian Sperm Transfer System (FAST®), 150–1, 154–5
fallopian tube patency, 1, 109–11
female factor infertility, *see* infertility
fertility counselling, *see* counselling
flare-up phenomenon, 67, 70
follicle stimulating hormone (FSH), 59–61
  recombinant, 60
  superovulation and, 81, 82, 87, 89
follicular development monitoring, 113–18

gamete intrafallopian transfer (GIFT), 24
  ovarian hyperstimulation syndrome and, 211
  pregnancy rates, 5
glycerol, as cryoprotectant, 165, 168, 195–6
gonadotrophin releasing hormone agonists (GnRHa), 2, 61–2
  insemination timing and, 83
  ovarian hyperstimulation syndrome and, 207, 211
  use in superovulation, 65–9, 83, 89
gonadotrophin releasing hormone (GnRH), 59, 61–2
gonadotrophins, 2, 60–1
  insemination timing and, 81–3
  ovarian hyperstimulation syndrome and, 207
  use in superovulation, 64–5
    sole use, 65, 88
    with clomiphene citrate, 64–5, 81–2, 86–7
    with GnRHa, 65–9, 83
growth hormone, adjunctive use of in superovulation, 69

health and safety, 18–19
human chorionic gonadotrophin (hCG), 2, 61, 113
  ovarian hyperstimulation syndrome and, 210–12
  timing of administration, 78–80
human menopausal gonadotrophin (hMG), 60
  superovulation and, 64, 81, 82, 86, 88
hydrosalpinges, 108–9
hypospadias, 28
hypospermia, 29
hysterosalpingo contrast sonography, 109–12

immunological infertility, 35–7, 227
implantation window, 119

impotence, 26–8
in vitro fertilization (IVF), 6–7, 90–1, 238
  clomiphene citrate therapy, 63–4
  counselling and, 52–3
  ovarian hyperstimulation syndrome and, 211
  poor follicular response to superovulation, 34
  pregnancy rates, 5
incubators, 12–14
infection, 222–5
infertility, 234–8
  female factor, 31–5
    allergy to semen, 34
    cervical factor, 32–3
    endometriosis, 34–5
    ovulatory dysfunction, 33–4
    vaginismus, 31
  immunological, 35–7, 227
  incidence, 234
  male factor, 24–31
    counselling and, 51
    ejaculatory dysfunction, 26–8
    highly viscous semen, 29–30
    hypospadias, 28
    hypospermia, 29
    impotence, 26–8
    retrograde ejaculation, 24–6
    subnormal sperm parameters, 30–1
  unexplained, 37
insemination, *see* intrauterine insemination
insemination room, 20
intracytoplasmic sperm injection (ICSI), 3, 178
intraperitoneal insemination (IPI), 5
intrauterine insemination (IUI), 1, 204, 238
  case summaries, 83–95
  complications of, 6
    allergic reactions, 226–7
    antisperm antibodies, 227
    ectopic pregnancy, 228–9
    infection, 222–5
    miscarriage, 228
    multiple pregnancy, 213–18
    non-infective salpingitis, 225–6
    ovarian hyperstimulation syndrome, 207–13
  indications for, 3–4
    with donor sperm, 40–1
    with fresh husband sperm, 24–37
    with frozen husband sperm, 37–40
  insemination methods, 2–3, 146–57
    conventional technique, 151–3
    Fallopian Sperm Transfer System (FAST®), 154–5
    Makler Insemination Device, 153–4
    post-insemination instructions, 155–7
  insemination timing, 79–83
    natural cycle, 81, 83–4
    with clomiphene citrate, 81, 85
    with clomiphene citrate and gonadotrophins, 81–2, 86–7
    with gonadotrophins, 82, 88
    with gonadotrophins and GnRHa, 83
  patient selection, 23–4
  success rates, 4–6

laparoscopy, 109–12
leiomyoma, uterine, 100–2
liquid nitrogen vapour, 180–1
live birth rates, 6
luteinising hormone (LH), 59–61
   LH surge, 62, 113
      in superovulation, 64–8, 78–83
      ovarian hyperstimulation syndrome and, 207–8
      ovulation timing and, 2, 78–81
      recombinant, 60–1
luteinising hormone-releasing hormone (LHRH), see gonadotrophin releasing hormone

Makler Insemination Device, 147–8, 153–4
male factor infertility, see infertility
Matheson-Carlborg-Gemzell medium, 176–7
microepididymal sperm aspiration, 3
miscarriage, 119, 228
Müllerian duct developmental defects, 99–100
multicultural issues, 53
multiple pregnancies, 2, 6, 70, 213–18

Nabothian follicles, 103
non-infective salpingitis, 225–6
nurses, 159–62
   administrative role, 162
   clinical role, 159–60
   counselling role, 161–2
   role in insemination, 160–1
nursing station, 20

oestrogen, 115
oligoasthenozoospermia, 30
oligospermia, 30
outpatient clinic facilities, 20
ovarian cancer, 70, 218–22
ovarian cysts
   superovulation and, 69–70, 105
   ultrasound diagnosis, 104–6
ovarian hyperstimulation syndrome, 2, 6, 7, 70, 118, 207–13
   case summary, 94
   polycystic ovarian syndrome and, 70, 107
   prevention of, 210–12
   treatment of, 212–13
ovarian stimulation, 2, 56
   follicular development monitoring, 113–18
   regimens, 78
   see also superovulation
ovulation:
   induction of, 56, 58
      pregnancy rates, 5
      side-effects of drugs, 208
   timing of, 2, 77–81
   ultrasound diagnosis of, 118
ovulatory dysfunction, 33–4

patient selection, 23–4
pelvic inflammatory disease, 109, 222–3, 228
Percoll gradients, 1, 3, 140
   non-infective salpingitis and, 225–6

percutaneous epididymal sperm aspiration, 3
polycystic ovarian syndrome:
   ovarian hyperstimulation syndrome and, 70, 107
   superovulation and, 60, 66, 69, 70
      case summaries, 92–4
   ultrasound diagnosis, 106–8
polyps, 103
polyvinyl alcohol (PVA), 196–7
pregnancy rates, 4–5
programmable freezing of human semen, 172, 181
protective clothing, 18–19
PureSperm, 140–4

religious issues, 53
retrograde ejaculation, 24–6
Rhesus isoimmunisation, 41, 202–4

salpingitis, 225–6
semen
   allergy to, 34, 226–7
   analysis of, 130–5
      staining technique, 133
   collection of, 129–30, 241
      collection room, 10–11
      for cryopreservation, 169–70, 174–5
      from donors, 195
      in irremediable impotence, 26, 28
   drug detrimental effects, 39–40
   highly viscous semen, 29–30
   organisms in, 222–4
   poor semen parameters, 39
   see also cryopreservation of semen; sperm
semenology facilities, 11–19
   consumables, 16–18
   hardware, 11–16
   health and safety, 18–19
   personnel, 11
sonography, see ultrasound scanning
sperm
   antisperm antibodies, 35–7, 227
   cryopreservation effects on, 182–3
      assessment of, 184–5
      sperm membranes, 165–7
      thawing effects on survival, 183
   malformations, 134
   morphological assessment, 131
   preparation of, 1, 2–3, 135–44
   subnormal sperm parameters, 30–1
   surgically recovered sperm, 3, 179
   see also donor sperm banking; semen
spontaneous abortion, 119, 228
straws, 179–80, 197
   removal from, 184
superovulation, 2, 56
   agents used, 57–62
      clomiphene citrate, 57–60, 63–4, 85
      clomiphene citrate and gonadotrophins, 64–5, 86–7
      GnRH and agonists, 61–2, 89
      gonadotrophins, 60–1, 65, 88
      gonadotrophins and GnRHa, 65–9
      growth hormone, adjunctive use, 69

case summaries, 85–95
complications of, 69–71, 207–22
   multiple pregnancies, 70, 213–18
   ovarian cancer, 70, 218–22
   ovarian hyperstimulation syndrome, 70, 207–13
follicular development monitoring, 113–18
methods, 62–9
monitoring, 62–3
ovarian cysts and, 69–70, 105
poor follicular response to, 34
surgically recovered sperm, 179

tamoxifen, 59–60
teratozoospermia, 30–1
testicular sperm extraction, 3
transvaginal sonography, 97–8
  *see also* ultrasound scanning
tubal patency, 1, 109–11
twin pregnancies, *see* multiple pregnancies

ultrasound scanning, 19–20, 97–9
   endometrial evaluation, 118–24
   follicular development monitoring, 113–18
   hysterosalpingo contrast sonography, 109–12
   ovulation diagnosis, 118
   ovulation timing, 78
   pelvic pathology diagnosis, 99–109
     endometriosis, 103–4
     hydrosalpinges, 108–9
     Müllerian duct developmental defects, 99–100
     Nabothian follicles, 103
     ovarian cysts, 104–6
     polycystic ovaries, 106–8
     polyps, 103
     uterine leiomyoma, 100–2
urine alkalisation, 25
uterine cancer, 220
uterine leiomyoma, 100–2

vaginal acidity, 1
vaginal bleeding, 95
vaginismus, 31
vapour freezing, 172, 181
vas deferens, congenital absence of, 3
vasectomy, 38

wash and swim-up sperm preparation technique, 1, 3, 137
  with PureSperm, 144